Healthy by Nature

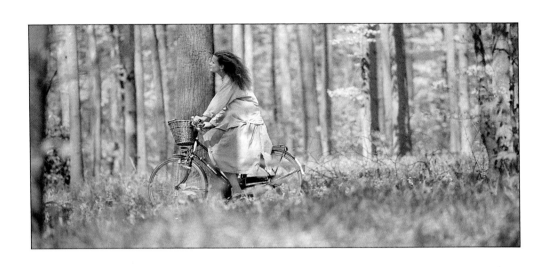

Healthy by Nature

Beth MacEoin

Thorsons
An Imprint of HarperCollins*Publishers*

Thorsons
An Imprint of HarperCollins*Publishers*
77–85 Fulham Palace Road
Hammersmith, London W6 8JB

First published by Thorsons 1994
1 3 5 7 9 10 8 6 4 2

Text illustrations by Andrea Norton

A catalogue record for this book
is available from the British Library

ISBN 0 7225 2803 5

Produced by HarperCollins Hong Kong

The information included in this book is advisory in
nature and does not form a substitute for professional
medical treatment, either orthodox or alternative.
Neither author nor publisher can accept responsibility
for the consequences of self-treatment or
unsupervised exercise.

For Denis, truly, madly, deeply.

Acknowledgements

Without the help, support and guidance of the following, this book would never have been written. My thanks go to my agent Teresa Chris who has given me as much help through moral support and a lively sense of humour as through practical suggestions. Thanks, also, to Eileen Campbell, Jane Graham-Maw and Rosemary Staheyeff at Thorsons.

Because the scope of this book is so wide, many people have been called on to offer advice, comments and suggestions on their relevant topics. Thanks are due to the alternative therapists who have given a large amount of assistance and advice on the 'Homoeopathy in Context' chapter. These include Norman Vaughton, Russel Dice, Penelope Ody, and Neil Thompson. My thanks go to Marion Bowles for taking a great deal of time to offer some excellent advice on the general content of the nutrition chapter; others who made valuable contributions within this section and to whom I also extend my thanks include Audrey Eyton, Doris Grant, Jean Joice, Tricia Millar, Leslie Kenton, Suzy Swanson and Michel Montignac.

The exercise chapter has also benefited from the expert advice of many people. These include Lesley Ackland, Lotte Berk, Carole Caplin, Lucy Jackson and Diana Kendall. Others who must be thanked for taking time out of very busy schedules to offer comments include Shirley Trickett for her constructive advice on the introductory and later chapters; Miranda Castro, who provided an extremely positive perspective on the chapter on homoeopathy for which I am very grateful; and Mary Clark, who took time to read the entire manuscript despite a heavy work schedule. Thanks are also due to Dr John Meldrum and Angela Morse for their suggestions and comments on Chapter Two.

My Mother Nancy must also be included: without her energy and strength of will my concept of vitality would probably be much less ambitious. Last, but not least, my thanks as always go to Denis and Sammy. The former because he is an unfailing source of positive encouragement, inspiration and practical advice on how to get out of a terrible mess with a word processor. The latter, just because he is who he is.

Photographs

Contents

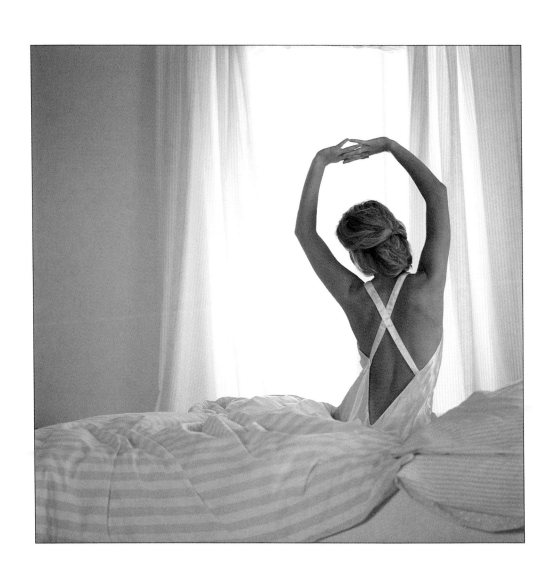

Introduction

Women are constantly receiving information about how to feel better, look wonderful, achieve more, and still look after the other people in their lives. While this can be instructive and inspiring, it can also be very confusing: many of us feel as though we are wandering through a maze of information full of the most contradictory advice.

Healthy by Nature has been written in order to clarify some of this information, cutting through anything that seems superfluous and concentrating on the essentials. As a result, I hope you will find the advice contained within simple, accessible, and—most important of all—achievable.

The reason this book is aimed at a female audience is simple: more and more in these emancipated days, we find ourselves performing a complex balancing act between time spent with family and children, time at work, and what little time we may have left for ourselves. Within this context we need all the help we can get from good nutrition to give us energy, exercise to diffuse stress, relaxation techniques to help us unwind, and an overall approach to health care that enhances our resilience.

This all sounds a tall order, and many of us have been put off attempting to incorporate these features in our lives because we don't know how or where to start. As a result, we end up feeling even more stressed and guilty.

In this book, I have aimed to put this daunting amount of information in perspective, giving the reader sound, practical advice on exercise, nutrition, alternative health care, and relaxation. How you choose to use this information is completely up to you. If you are interested in health matters as a whole you will want to read the book from cover to cover; if you are especially interested in nutrition or exercise you may want to concentrate on those sections and just dip into others; and if your main interest lies in alternative medicine you may choose to read the chapter on homoeopathy and other therapies first.

This is essentially a book about change: the sort of change that enables us to see that we can aim for a more balanced way of life that may have seemed beyond our grasp. The first step is to have as wide a picture of health, fitness, and well-being as possible and then, bit by bit, to start putting the different elements together in our own lives.

Please look upon the material in this book as friendly advice. Above all, never feel guilty or despairing if you can't achieve everything you aim to do at first: change takes time and we all have the feeling occasionally of taking one step forward and two steps back.

The main thing is to keep on going. Before long, you will begin to see that once you have started to make positive changes to your lifestyle, the commitment and energy you need to go further will become available to you. As your sense of well-being increases, so will your energy levels and, in turn, your self-esteem. By taking a first step on this path you will be assuming responsibility for your own health.

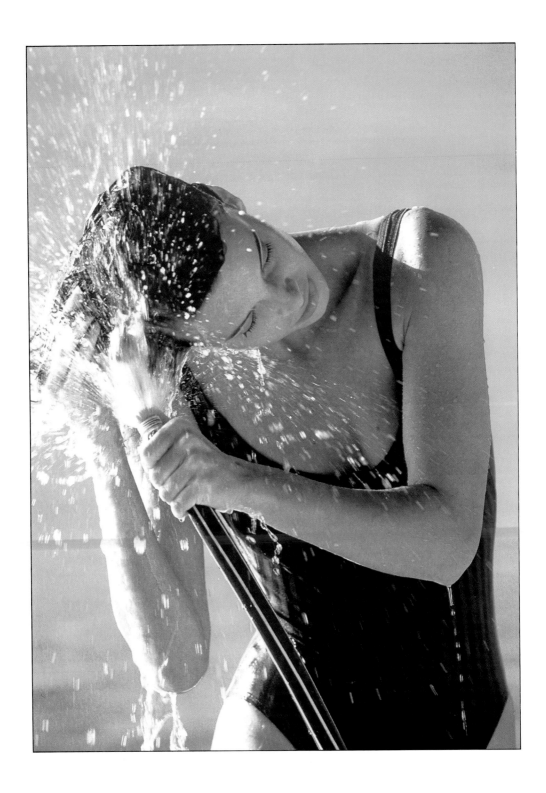

CHAPTER ONE

Pathways To Health

What is Positive Health?

Positive health is quite different from what most of us have grown accustomed to. It is more then the mere absence of illness, more than being free of symptoms; it's about having an abundance of energy, vitality, and enthusiasm for life. This abundance is the absolute opposite of what many of us feel much of the time: lethargic, jaded, and exhausted to the point where everyday demands become impossible to meet.

Of course, even when we enjoy positive health, there will always be times when life is just too stressful, demanding, or depressing. This isn't a book about miracles! The difference is that when we work from the baseline of positive health, our resilience and capacity for recovery are much greater than when we are experiencing chronic fatigue, lethargy and overall poor health. When we feel down, the struggle to cope from one day to the next can become a bleak downward spiral that seems impossible to break. But it needn't be

that way. With positive health, every new day can be a step on the road to energy, fulfilment and vitality.

If you are worried that achieving all of this will mean giving up your friends and everyday pleasures, think again. The path to positive health does not lie through self-punishment and self-denial. A spartan approach involving exercise you find boring, a diet that is uninspiring, or a lifestyle that is too rigid, can end up leaving you uninspired and guilt-ridden. Obviously, some basic positive changes in attitude or routine will help you to achieve and maintain good health. But this needn't involve you in constant self-examination. On the contrary, experiencing positive health will give you the zest and vitality to expand your interests and enhance the quality of your experience of life, rather than diminishing it.

Taking Responsibility

Until comparatively recently, the quality of our health has been regarded by many of us as something for which we have very little responsibility, and over which we have equally little control. This abdication of responsibility has led to a potentially disastrous combination: the overuse of prescription drugs and a tendency to feel distanced from our own bodies. The more we have lost touch with how our bodies feel when they function at an optimum level, the less capable we are of identifying problems as they arise. This can lead us to ignore continually the subtle messages our bodies are sending us, telling us that all is not well, until things progress to a point where it is impossible to ignore the problems any longer because they are becoming increasingly disabling.

Problems with the 'Quick Fix' Approach

By the time things have reached this stage, the 'quick fix' or 'magic bullet' approach may temporarily ease the situation for us, and we tend to presume that this approach to medicine is the only one available to us. Unfortunately, this approach encourages us to think of our bodies as no more than machines that need the odd spare part from time to time. It is this way of thinking that leads us to talk about going to the doctor's surgery for our MOT or ten thousand mile service. While this may be fine on one level, it leads us unwittingly towards a reliance on drugs which are targeted to specific systems of our bodies, and ultimately to 'spare-part' surgery.

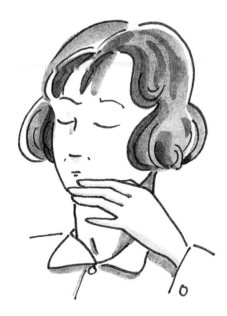

If we follow this course without attending to the underlying imbalances in our overall health, the chances are that we will just find the same problems recurring. Instead of relying on the 'quick fix', therefore, we need to learn to see the broader picture: that of our body as an integrated whole, that is in turn part of the greater wholeness of mind, body and spirit.

A Balanced Perspective

We are increasingly aware that there are more contributory factors to disease than exposure to viruses, bacteria or cancer-causing agents. Of course these play their part, but not everyone who is subjected to these factors will contract a disease. If we enjoy positive health then our minds and bodies are in optimum balance, and our immune systems or defence mechanisms are better equipped to deal with any invading agents of disease.

In other words, what we are dealing with is a two-way process: the state of health we are in when we are exposed to infections matters as much as, if not more than, the fact of exposure itself.

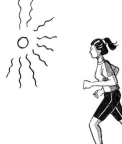

Ways of Pursuing the Path of Positive Fitness

- Work in harmony with your body, developing a keen sense of which elements in your life cause negative stress, and those which maximize your energy potential and sense of well-being.

- Begin to see your mind and body as a dynamic, integrated whole, responding continually to factors around you. Be aware that your health is not a static entity, but fluctuates both positively and negatively to factors in your environment.

- Be aware of warning signs when they appear, however undramatic they may appear at first. They may be no more than symptoms of a minor skin condition that refuses to clear, recurring infections, changes in our menstrual cycle, or just plain tiredness. If we ignore these signs we may be storing up more problems, since these symptoms are the mechanism our bodies have for communicating to us that all is not well. If we take positive action at this stage, we can avoid a worsening of the situation, and improve our potential for good health.

Alternative Medicine and the Concept of Positive Health

The major systems of alternative medicine such as homoeopathy, acupuncture, herbalism and osteopathy all work from the basic premise that our bodies and minds make up an integrated whole. In good health, our bodies function smoothly to the extent that attention is not drawn to any single part by the warning signal of pain. Once symptoms begin to appear, it is a sign that all is not well within our systems; if they persist, we will need treatment to restore the smooth functioning of our bodies. The treatment will vary from therapy to therapy, but each has in common with the others the basic concept of reinforcing our in-built capacity to heal ourselves, rather than simply suppressing symptoms.

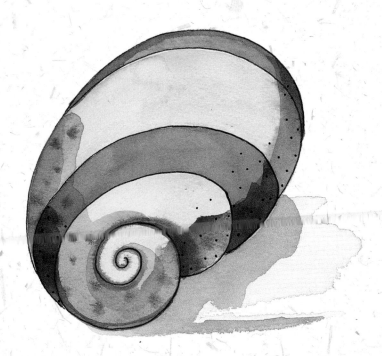

The Importance of a Holistic Approach

The therapies mentioned above are all examples of alternative approaches which employ a holistic approach. Holistic treatments will:

- Concern themselves with the smooth functioning of our bodies as a whole, rather than with the specific malfunctioning of certain areas in isolation. From a holistic point of view, it is as necessary to enquire into someone's mental and emotional experience since ill health began, as it is to ask for details of the physical problem.

- Promote the idea that there is a wide range of specific physical disorders that are linked to our state of mind and emotional well-being. Good examples would include migraine, irritable bowel syndrome, and hypertension. Although orthodox doctors are increasingly seeing links between these diseases and stress reactions, a holistic therapist would go further and see conditions such as arthritis, eczema, and menstrual disorders as frequently being physical expressions of emotional stress and trauma, which may either be ongoing or have their roots in the past; or that these conditions result from combined physical, mental and emotional imbalances.

- Avoid assessing the quality of our health purely on the basis of symptom removal, by taking into consideration the day-to-day quality of our life and well-being.

The Importance of Prevention

A holistic system of health care such as homoeopathy is especially appropriate when used within the context of preventative medicine. In other words, it is totally in order to consult a homoeopath either when we are in reasonable health and want to improve its quality further, or when early non-specific symptoms have arisen such as persistent tiredness, muscle aches and pains, or recurrent infections, which indicate that we may be at risk of further decline.

In other words, because homoeopathy is a system of healing that is more concerned with the enhancement our general levels of health and vitality than with the simple removal of symptoms it is an especially appropriate model of health care to consider in any discussion of the merits of positive health.

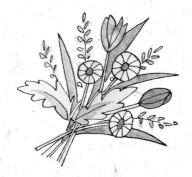

What we are essentially concerned with here is how to elevate our experience of health and well-being to the point where it makes a qualitative difference to our perception of day-to-day living. It is very hard to feel enthusiastic about either work or leisure when energy levels are down to zero on a daily basis, or when we are plagued by recurrent minor infections. A medical system such as homoeopathy, in common with other holistic therapies, works by giving our bodies a much needed energy boost so that its own curative potential can be released. It can also provide the added bonus of releasing additional energy which we can put to creative use.

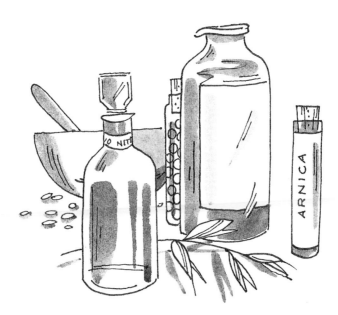

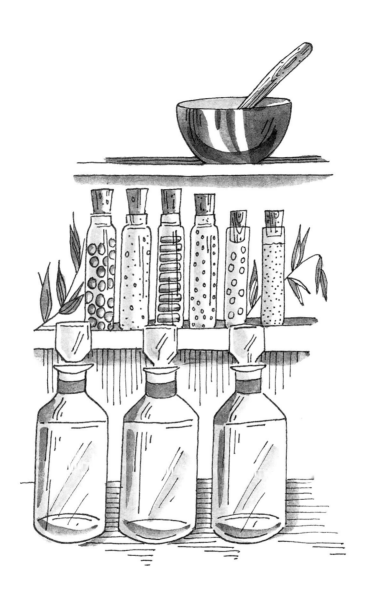

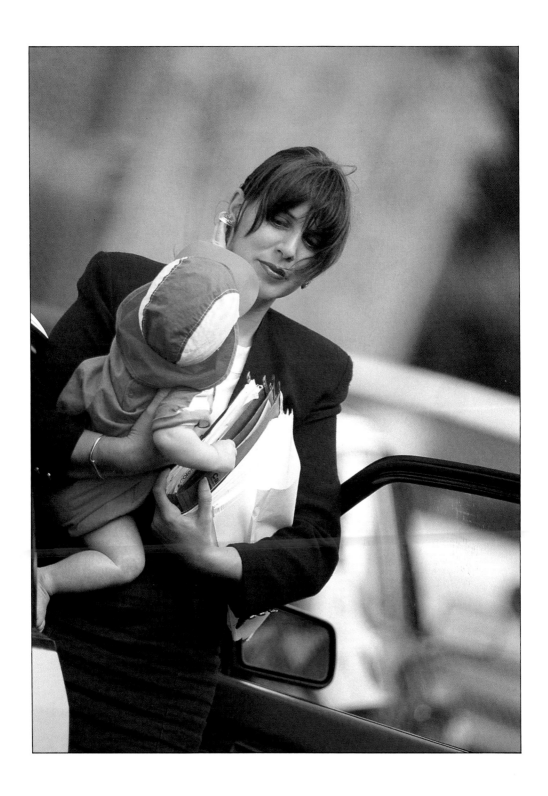

CHAPTER TWO

Limitations to Health

A Fresh Perspective

If we want to enhance our experience of health rather than limit ourselves to treating illnesses when they arrive, we need to look for additional help beyond current orthodox medical measures. The reason why this is so is simple: modern medicine emphasizes the treatment of symptoms rather than ways of enhancing and supporting our experience of health.

Although there are situations that modern medicine is excellently suited to deal with, there are others where orthodox drugs or surgery may be unable to improve the overall quality of our health. Examples of the positive aspects of orthodox medicine include:

- Diagnosis of life-threatening condtions.

- Emergency surgery.

- Intervention in severe, acute episodes of illness such as meningitis.

- First-aid situations where a fracture or severe bleeding has occurred.

- Surgery that enables us to regain mobility, such as hip replacement operations.

- Situations that require strong pain relief or anaesthesia.

Even here, patients may be considerably helped by the judicious use of alternative methods both during and after treatment.

Problems with the Mechanical Approach to Health

Although orthodox medicine is excellent at dealing with the situations mentioned above, there are other conditions that pose more of a problem. These are the less dramatic, more long-term health problems such as asthma, acne, eczema, painful periods, pre-menstrual syndrome, depression, or arthritis. Reasons for the difficulty in treating these long-term, chronic conditions are linked to:

- The emphasis that orthodox medicine places on the removal or suppression of symptoms, rather than attempting to deal with the underlying imbalance which may be causing the problem. As a result, the best results that can be obtained are those which provide short-term relief.

- Orthodox medicine's concern with the external trigger for disease, rather than with ways of supporting the self-healing abilities of our bodies. Although this can be of enormous value in supplying information of a 'cause and effect' nature, it has major limitations when it is applied as the *only* explanation of disease.

- The classification of symptoms into separate categories, all of which require different treatments. Because of this high degree of specialization, investigative tests have become increasingly invasive. This can leave us feeling frightened and frustrated if our symptoms refuse to fit into the framework of the appropriate test.

An added problem which relates to over-specialization is the concept of the human body as a machine which can be broken down into component parts to be repaired or replaced when necessary. This does not encourage us to see the essential links between our minds, emotions and bodies, or to explore ways of supporting our health through positive changes in our social and working environment, or in our eating patterns.

- Orthodox medicine's lack of investigation into the question of susceptibility. In other words, why is it that, in a 'flu epidemic, some of us fall ill while others can resist the infection? We may all have been exposed to the same virus, but our responses to the virus will differ according to our own level of health and vitality at that time.

The Body/Mind Link

If we take seriously the idea of susceptibility to illness we have to consider the essential importance of external factors operating on our bodies. These may include:

- Emotional stress.

- Financial strain.

- Physical strain such as unreasonably long and stressful hours of work.

- Bad eating habits, perhaps because of extra pressure.

- Reliance on stimulants such as coffee, alcohol or cigarettes to keep going.

As you can imagine, we could extend this list much further if we looked at all of the varied factors which lead us to feel stressed on mental, emotional and physical levels.

The importance of taking our stress levels into account is becoming increasingly relevant, as evidence accumulates that the amount of stress we experience and how we choose to deal with it can have a profound effect on the function of our immune systems. Since we are dependent on the healthy and vigorous functioning of our immune systems in order to maintain optimum fitness, the condition of our immune functioning is crucial to any discussion of positive health.

Grief and Depression of our Immune Systems

Studies conducted at New York's Mount Sinai Hospital School of Medicine in the late 1970s revealed that depression of our immune systems can follow from experiences of sadness and grief. Other disorders such as hardening of the arteries, high blood pressure, and problems with our digestion can all be considered reactions of the body to stressful stimuli. Most important of all, it is now apparent that it is our individual reactions to stressful situations that determine whether or not they will take their toll on our bodies and minds. The good news is that we can turn this knowledge to our advantage by taking steps to protect and stimulate our immune systems in a positive direction through a combination of relaxation techniques, meditation, exercise, and diet.

This obviously takes us beyond the search for the specific disease agent to a holistic philosophy that stresses the mind-body spectrum and the importance of individual susceptibility and resistance. By making this fresh start, we will soon find ourselves exploring ideas outside the limited range of what is considered possible by conventional medical science. Once we do that, there is no end to the exciting possibilities in front of us.

The Concept of the 'Magic Bullet'

We are all familiar with the idea of the 'magic bullet' which is specifically targeted to eliminating a problem situation in our bodies: many advertisements make use of such imagery in their campaigns to sell pain-killers or decongestants. None of us can deny the attraction of such an image, which conveys strength, power, speed and precision; but sadly, evidence suggests that, as always, nothing in life is that simple.

Problems associated with the 'magic bullet' approach to treatment include potentially damaging side effects, drug dependency, and the loss of the essential truth that prevention is better than cure.

Side Effects

The intention behind the 'magic bullet' was to develop a treatment which would be targeted to destroy a specific disease-producing agent in our bodies, leaving other areas unaffected. Sadly, experience has taught us that this has not been possible. Drugs will constantly interact with what we eat or drink, or with other drugs that we may be taking. They may also produce unpleasant side-effects or possible allergic reactions.

But on an even more profound level, we have to question whether it is possible to achieve an alteration in the chemical balance of one bodily system without provoking sympathetic changes in another. We are all familiar with the downward spiral in which someone is given a specific drug to treat one group of symptoms; this gives rise to side-effects elsewhere needing separate drug treatment, and so on and on, the complications growing with each drug administered. Many of us will have experienced a straightforward example of this process in taking repeated courses of antibiotics for cystitis, which have been followed closely by digestive disorders or thrush demanding separate treatment.

Drug Dependence

The 'magic bullet' approach attempts to suppress or attack the disease agent in isolation from other bodily systems and does not support our bodies in doing the job for themselves. As a result, we can be left needing to take drugs on a long-term basis—because the fundamental

imbalance in our body, which produced the symptoms in the first place, has not been addressed.

Extra problems also arise when we take into account how psychological and physiological factors interact to make us dependent. If we take the example of tranquillizers, once we have become physiologically dependent, we can experience severe and distressing symptoms if we try to reduce or stop taking the tablets. If we have also become psychologically dependent the situation can be even more difficult to manage, as it becomes increasingly difficult for us to unravel which of our symptoms relate to panic about the withholding of a course of drugs, and what is a straightforward physical reaction to withdrawal.

Loss Of An Integrated Vision Of Our Bodies

Perhaps most disturbing of all, the logical result of treatment by 'magic bullet' is a loss of perspective. When we suffer illness, it may not necessarily be limited to one specific area, but can be much more diffused and widespread. If we lose sight of this fact, there is a danger that we will expect medical treatment to provide nothing more than localized symptom removal. Once this has happened, we are left with a medical system which is essentially concerned with sickness management and which is unlikely to encourage us to improve the quality of health by ourselves.

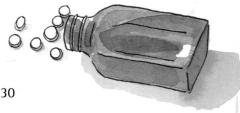

Unfortunately, the reliance on the 'magic bullet' has led us to assume that there is 'a pill for every ill', and that we need not take steps in the early stages of ill health, since our symptoms can be removed by taking a drug if they persist or worsen later on. It is this line of thinking that has left many of us divorced from our own state of health, often feeling helpless when illness does strike because we have abdicated responsibility for the state of our bodies to the medical profession. The 'magic bullet' does little to encourage us to see the quality of our health as something that can be supported and enhanced by fundamental changes in our lifestyle.

Women and Orthodox Medical Care

As women we come into regular contact with orthodox medicine at central stages of development in our lives. Experiencing major life events such as puberty, pregnancy, and the menopause can often lead us to the doctor's surgery in search of help.

Although orthodox medicine has developed and refined its approach to treatment since the last century, some tensions and dissatisfactions remain for women when it comes to drug therapy and surgery. Many of us are frustrated by the lack of help available for conditions such as PMS (Pre-Menstrual Syndrome) or painful periods. Little advice may be forthcoming beyond the recommendation of painkillers or diuretics, which can leave us feeling helpless and unsure of where to look for further help. We can also experience a dilemma when faced with a choice with regard to treatment about which we may feel unable to make an informed decision, such as Hormone Replacement Therapy.

Since our menstrual cycles are especially reactive to stress, with irregularities following on from emotional or physical trauma, it makes good sense to explore symptoms beyond the purely physical level in these situations. This does not suggest that we are not suffering from real symptoms and that the problem is 'all in the mind'. On the contrary, these conditions are accompanied by distressing, debilitating and disabling sensations all of which are emphatically physical, but we have a far greater chance of experiencing a favourable outcome if we are seen as a person operating in, and reacting to, situations that are unique to us.

Signs of Change

Although it is now likely that if we suffer from PMS we will have the option of being referred to a PMS clinic, this does not necessarily mean that we have a better chance of receiving more holistic treatment. Some clinics offer dietary advice, and some recommend the use of supplements such as Evening Primrose Oil or Vitamin B_6, or they may suggest using the hormone progesterone.

While some of these measures may improve symptoms considerably (in trials

31

at St Thomas's Hospital in London, over 60 per cent of women experienced relief of symptoms using Evening Primrose Oil), treatment along these lines is still concerned with symptom relief rather than attempting to rectify the underlying imbalance which led to the condition. It is also worth saying that hard evidence for the effectiveness of Evening Primrose Oil in treating PMS is yet to be forthcoming, and that one recent trial concluded that a paraffin oil placebo could be equally effective in relieving symptoms.

Taking a vitamin supplement may feel more satisfying than swallowing a diuretic, since it seems closer to a natural source; but on its own this is not a move towards a more holistic approach. This will only be the case if the supplement is combined with a broader assessment of general lifestyle and well-being. Used within this broader context, the supplementary approach can have a helpful and positive part to play in restoring us to good health.

Childbirth and Medicine

Many women become aware of the problems involved in a mechanical approach to medicine when we experience pregnancy and childbirth. For many of us, this will be the first time that we are subjected to a wide range of tests and investigative procedures, and it is all too easy to lose sight of the psychological impact of the experience in the midst of medical practices which can leave us feeling lost and anxious. This

anxiety can be increased for us if we choose to have our first baby in our thirties or forties: falling into a high-risk category inevitably brings uncertainties, feelings which can be heightened by tests such as amniocentesis, which have their own controversial problems.

High-Tech Versus Minimal Intervention

It would be absurd to suggest that medical intervention is redundant or unnecessary in childbirth; but when a high-tech approach is applied with excessive zeal it can cause problems of its own. In The Netherlands, the incidence of infant mortality and birth trauma is impressively low, especially when compared to Britain and America. And yet, in The Netherlands medical intervention in pregnancy and labour is kept to a minimum, and a positive emphasis is put on home births. Professional midwives are an important source of care during labour, whether the birth takes place at home or in hospital. It appears that when they are too enthusiastically applied, high-tech procedures can and do cause problems that are avoided by adopting a responsible low-tech approach.

If we use labour and childbirth as a model for alternative ways of approaching a medicine, we can see how the perspective could be changed. We could improve the experience of birth for many women by providing simple advice on diet and relaxation to help mothers with a tendency to high blood pressure, by employing TENS machines, hypnotherapy or acupuncture for pain relief, and using homoeopathy to ensure good health during pregnancy and as a means of easing the stages of labour.

By broadening out the possibilities in this way, we could envisage a situation where high-tech procedures could be used to maximum advantage in situations that demand more urgent and radical intervention, while taking second place to gentler methods in more normal circumstances.

In fact, advances along these lines have already been made in some places, since in some hospitals it is possible for a mother who is keen to use non-orthodox measures during labour to avail herself of a more natural form of childbirth and pain relief, provided she has the consent of her consultant.

Further Possibilities

If we expand this model and look at general health problems from the same perspective, we can see that equally exciting possibilities are open to us. In other words, instead of opting immediately for an antibiotic as the first resort, there are a number of other potential treatments available, which span the range from judicious use of homoeopathy in order to deal with the acute infection to more long-term strategies such as constitutional homoeopathic prescribing, acupuncture, dietary advice, or herbal therapy. We may still choose to opt for antibiotic treatment in the end, but if this is done after

considering other options this is much more positive than just assuming that the only available option is an orthodox drug.

Exciting developments along these lines have already begun, such as the establishment of Britain's first NHS clinic offering complementary therapies at Marylebone, London. In this clinic orthodox doctors work with alternative practitioners offering acupuncture, homoeopathy, massage, or healing to patients. Other health centres around Britain are increasingly making use of the services of alternative therapists, and a recent survey suggested that 80 per cent of GPs considered homoeopathy to be effective. In the same survey, 43 per cent were willing to refer patients to homoeopathic practitioners while 79 per cent wanted homoeopathy to be included in regular medical tuition.

Before we can consider the appropriateness of an alternative therapy for ourselves we need to have enough information to guide us in making our choice. The information in the next two chapters will give you a broad idea of the possibilities open to you.

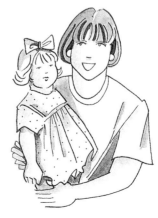

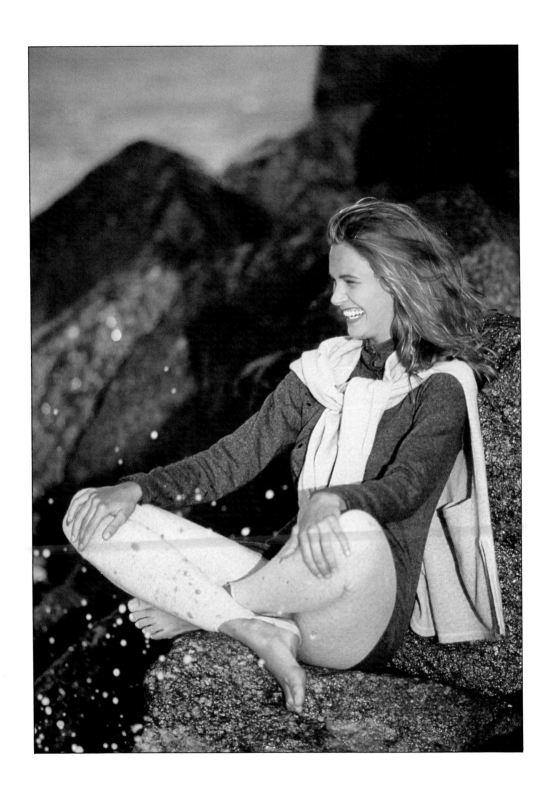

CHAPTER THREE

The Homoeopathic Approach:
Achieving the Balance

A New Model of Health Care

It is clear that many people today are searching for an approach to medical care that reflects their growing preoccupation with holistic approaches to living. As concern for the well-being of the planet grows, more and more us are also becoming involved in caring for our own physical and emotional well-being.

From this perspective, traditional approaches to health care will seem out of step. Using a 'magic bullet' to zap the invading bacterium without taking into account the effect of the drug on our organisms as a whole is clearly unsatisfactory. Increasingly large numbers of us are waking up to the fact that relying on pills to maintain a mediocre level of health is not enough—we need to play a more active role if we are to achieve optimum health and vitality.

It is noticeable that women feature strongly in this move towards a broader concept of health care, whether in their capacity as carers within their families, in a professional context as complementary practitioners, or simply as women desiring to take responsibility for their own health. Qualities traditionally associated with women, such as caring, capacity for reflection, and nurturing, clearly come into their own in alternative approaches to medicine, where the individual is considered as a whole and efforts are made to integrate his or her physical, mental, and emotional aspects.

What is Homoeopathy?

Homoeopathy is an independent system of medicine that has existed for almost two hundred years. It is practised by both doctors trained in orthodox medicine and professional homoeopaths on a world-wide basis, and is one of the most popular forms of complementary medicine available today.

The Concept of Similars

The word 'homoeopathy' literally means 'similar suffering'. In other words, a substance which can cause symptoms of illness in a healthy person can be used as a curative agent in cases of illness where the same symptoms have appeared. In cases of Arsenic poisoning, for example, we would expect to see symptoms of severe vomiting, diarrhoea, chills, and tremendous restlessness. However, these are also common symptoms of food poisoning, and, not surprisingly, Arsenic (*Arsenicum album*) is one of the most frequently indicated homoeopathic remedies in such cases (considerably diluted, of course!). Where the symptoms of the remedy picture and those of the sick person match, the body's capacity for self-healing is activated and symptoms can be resolved at all levels.

The idea of treating illness through using similar substances had existed from the time of Hippocrates, but Samuel Hahnemann (1755–1843), the founder of modern homoeopathy, developed the basic concept into a fully fledged and powerful medical system. In exploring his ideas about sickness and health, he opposed the conventional doctors of his day, who insisted on prescribing drugs to suppress symptoms of illness, thus having an 'opposite' effect and rarely, if ever, curing the patient.

The Concept of Provings

In order to establish what medicinal effects a substance would have on a healthy person, Hahnemann carried out a series of controlled experiments on himself and other volunteers. These experiments were called 'provings' and involved the regular administration of a substance, with effects being recorded. Volunteers for provings had to be in good health and free of any symptoms which might mask the results. They also had to record in meticulous detail any changes in their emotional and physical health for the duration of the experiment.

The same principles apply today, since hundreds of remedies in use have been proved in this way, and new remedies are added as more provings are carried out.

The Minimum Dose

As Hahnemann developed the concept of similar prescribing, he also experimented with using progressively smaller doses in order to avoid toxic effects. He had been sensitized to the distressing nature of drug reactions in patients during his training as an orthodox physician, and kept on diluting medicinal substances until he reached a point where he parted company with orthodox science.

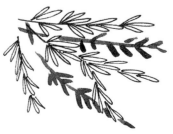

Although he was working at a level where no molecules of the original substance could be detected, Hahnemann found that these very dilute substances had a profound effect in stimulating a self-healing process in the body provided they were also subjected to an additional process of shaking or 'succussion' at each stage of dilution. Contrary to what one would expect, Hahnemann found that the further away he got from a material dose, the more powerful the medicinal effect proved to be—as long as there was still a marked similarity between the patient's symptoms and the medicine prescribed.

The Importance of Individualizing Symptoms

In order to establish a match between the relevant homoeopathic remedy and the patient's symptoms, homoeopaths have to gather considerably more information than the average G.P. or hospital specialist. Unlike most doctors they are not particularly interested in common symptoms.

In other words, in a case of severe cold, you would expect almost everyone to have symptoms common to the condition: a runny nose, sneezing fits, and a cough. But if you begin to enquire more carefully you may find that one person experiences a scanty, burning, clear nasal discharge, has a dry, wheezy cough which is much worse at night, and has felt unusually anxious since the onset of the cold,

while another person with the 'same' cold may have a thick, bland, green nasal discharge, with a cough that feels very loose on waking, and may have felt very weepy since falling ill.

As you can see, both people have been exposed to infection and have fallen ill in broadly the same way; but each one experiences individual symptoms which demonstrate their own particular response to being unwell. In the first case, the homoeopathic remedy *Arsenicum album* would match the symptoms well, while the second person would need a homoeopathic preparation called *Pulsatilla*. This is because it is the sick individual who is being prescribed for, not an abstract disease category called 'the common cold'.

Why Homoeopathic Treatment is Wonderful for Women

The numerous and often conflicting demands made on women are quite remarkable. At times it seems impossible to perform a delicate balancing act between the demands of a career, running a home, coping with motherhood, caring for other family members, finding time for a social life, or making space in which to relax. Given these demands, it makes sense for us to opt for a system of medicine that not only deals effectively with the symptoms of illness if they arise, but also strengthens our individual constitutions, and boosts our energy levels. Because homoeopathic treatment is able to support our bodies and work in harmony with responses to emotional or physical trauma, the potential benefits available to women from this form of therapy are enormous.

The Importance of the Whole Person

It is one of the major advantages for women receiving homoeopathic treatment that the practitioner is required to obtain a detailed picture of the quality of health experienced by patients as individuals on emotional, mental and physical levels. If we consider how many conditions affecting women not only have physical symptoms, but also effect profound changes in the emotional sphere, and that these are themselves often inextricably linked with physical disorders, any treatment which takes into account the effect of illness on the whole person is bound to be more gratifying and rewarding than one that does not.

By choosing to use homoeopathic medicine, it is possible for us to avoid the fragmented treatment that so often accompanies the use of orthodox drugs. Take the example of PMS: instead of taking diuretics for water retention, tranquillizers for mood swings, and a potassium supplement to make up for the mineral which is lost as a result of taking diuretics, a homoeopath will tailor a prescription

to the needs of our individual constitutions. Because there is time for the practitioner to put together a detailed case history including physical and emotional problems, we have a chance to identify patterns or inter-connecting factors that have not been seen before. Within this context it is possible to see that far more is involved here than removal of symptoms through the temporary action of drugs. This is one of the most fundamental steps we can take in the pursuit of positive health.

The Essential Connection Between Feeling Good and Looking Good

Any woman knows that when her energy levels are high and she is enjoying a sense of well-being, her skin tends to be clearer, her hair shinier, and her eyes more sparkling. When good health is experienced it is always outwardly visible. The reverse, of course, is also true. There is little point in spending a fortune in skin-care creams and make-up if all they can do is paste over the cracks.

Feeling and looking our best is not confined to how others see us, it is also intimately linked to how confident we feel about ourselves. If we look in the mirror and see a lack-lustre face with puffy eyes with bags underneath them the size of suitcases, it is very hard to feel convinced that we have the zest and vitality to meet the demands of the day. If we reverse the picture, feeling good about ourselves is contagious:

once we feel positive and confident we become more resilient and less demoralized by criticism. Feeling positive is dependent on having a zest for life, and this in turn depends on how much vital energy a person has.

We can all think of days when going out and having fun seems too much of a bother because our energy levels are down to almost zero. On the other hand, when these levels are high, the most tiresome and unexciting tasks seem within reach, and things just fall into place. In both these scenarios, the surrounding context can be the same: it is the way the individual feels about herself and the world that has changed. If a system of health care is chosen which supports the energizing, cleansing, eliminating, and renewing properties of the body, and if this is combined with basic dietary advice and regular exercise, we can take the first steps to reaching a state of improved harmony between mind and body. A holistic approach to treatment is not a magic wand: all the usual problems which are part and parcel of life will still be there; but it will offer a wider range of strategies with which to deal with them.

Problems With Side-Effects

When we choose to use an alternative medical system in conjunction with relaxation techniques, massage, aromatherapy, and expert advice on eating and exercise, this provides the basis for a sound and rewarding approach to caring for our minds and bodies. By opting for a system of health care such as homoeopathy, we can benefit from a therapy which avoids the side-effects and other pitfalls of orthodox drugs. For example, long-term reliance on steroid creams can cause the thinning and discolouration of the skin, while routine use of low-dosage antibiotics for treating acne will only have a temporary effect at best, and may lead to problems with recurring bouts of the yeast overgrowth we call thrush.

Most important of all, the best that orthodox drugs will provide will be short-term relief, or the suppression of symptoms. This is why many of us have been in the unhappy position of needing to take repeated courses of drugs in order to keep ourselves relatively symptom-free. If we look at a more holistic approach to medical care, we shall see that a system of healing such as homoeopathy, in common with other major systems such as acupuncture, will be searching to identify where the imbalance lies in our constitutional make-up which led to our ill health in the first place. By improving our overall quality of health, it is possible for symptoms to be resolved by the body itself, rendering long and repeated courses of drug therapy unnecessary because our bodies have regained a state of balance and internal harmony.

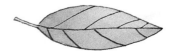

It would be naive and unrealistic to suggest that we discard orthodox drugs in their entirety: there are situations where emergency treatment with antibiotics or steroids will save lives. In many cases, however, orthodox drugs are ineffective or unsuitable for long-term treatment of chronic disorders.

This leads us to the possibility of a radical reorientation of our approach to health care: if we initially adopt a holistic approach in treating long-term problems such as acne, eczema, arthritis, and digestive problems, this could become an extremely effective first resort. The more heroic drugs such as steroids, anti-inflammatories, or antibiotics could then be reserved for the situations in which they are most effective, thus avoiding the increase of superbugs which refuse to respond to broad-spectrum antibiotics and other immensely powerful drugs.

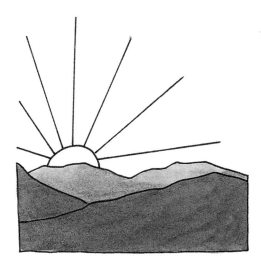

The Holistic Approach

A truly holistic medical system is one that is concerned with the individual and how that individual expresses their own particular disorder on the mental, emotional and physical levels.

Accustomed as we are to living life at a frantic pace, it is very easy to live as though we are only disembodied minds, and to forget to care for our bodies. Or the reverse may happen: we spend hours working out in the gym, only to find that we fail to give our minds time and space in which to relax. Equally, we can look after our minds and bodies very well, but forget that we also have emotional needs which are illogical and seem downright confusing if consistently neglected or ignored.

Only when all three levels are in harmony and in the optimum balance for us, can we achieve and maintain a dynamic state of positive health. This state of harmony will of course fluctuate in response to daily stimuli, but if serious disruption and long-term trauma disrupt this delicate balance, positive health becomes frustratingly elusive.

One of the most exciting aspects of a holistic treatment is the voyage of self-discovery on which we embark when responsibility is put into our hands. Undergoing homoeopathic treatment, for example, does not involve just a passive taking of pills, but requires us to become more in tune with our bodies and to register changes which take place during treatment. Broader advice will often be given on what aspects of our lifestyle may be hindering positive results, and what positive changes would speed up recovery. In this way, treatment involves the communication of information which can give us major insights with regard to our health problems and how we may unwittingly have contributed to them. This self-awareness is a vital tool in dissipating the feelings of helplessness we often associate with feeling unwell.

Current Alternative Medical Systems

There are many forms of alternative treatment now available, ranging from complete therapeutic systems such as acupuncture, herbalism and homoeopathy, to therapies that may be used in a more supportive, adjunctive, or 'complementary' context such as massage, shiatsu, iridology, osteopathy, naturopathy or reflexology. This range of options could be expanded to include systems like the Alexander Technique, Yoga, Feldenkrais, Dance Therapy, and many more.

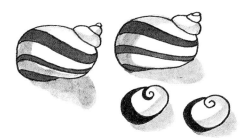

Homoeopathy is an excellent example of an alternative medical system which endeavours to treat us on mental, emotional and physical levels in an attempt to raise our overall experience of health and well-being. It shares, in common with other alternative therapies such as acupuncture, the basic philosophy that good health is more than the absence of disease, and that medical treatment should not be involved with mere symptom suppression.

Homoeopathy can be applied as a full therapeutic system for a range of disorders. On a preventative level it can be used as constitutional treatment enhancing energy levels and overall vitality and modifying inherited weaknesses. In pregnancy and childbirth it can be used to great effect in improving the overall health of mother and baby; it can also be invaluable as an aid to speeding up healing and recovery after surgery. In acute infectious illness, astute prescribing of homoeopathic remedies can speed up recovery and avoid complications, and in states of emotional trauma and shock, sedation can be provided without complications or side effects.

This gives just a limited insight into the potential scope of homoeopathy as a medical system. In the following sections we shall see how it is an excellent model for a holistic form of health care fully appropriate to the needs of today.

41

What Can I Expect On A First Visit To A Homoeopath?

~

When you consult a homoeopath for the first time be prepared for a lengthy first appointment. An average initial consultation usually takes about one and a half hours. You may think this sounds a daunting period of time to spend with a health professional, but you will be surprised how quickly the time passes once the consultation gets underway.

On the first visit you will need to convey basic information regarding your current state of health, present and past symptoms, a detailed medical history including diseases suffered by your family and relatives, and information regarding any drugs that you have taken.

Most important of all, your homoeopath will need to gain as broad a picture as possible of what makes you tick on the mental and emotional levels. In doing so, you may find that she asks unusual questions. She may, for example, try to discover what reactions you have to atmospheric changes, or what time of day you feel at your best or your worst. The reason behind this questioning is quite straightforward: it is only by asking very detailed questions about your reactions to your daily surroundings that your homoeopath can begin to build up a picture of how you respond to situations as an individual.

The purpose behind this gathering of information is to enable your homoeopath to gain as accurate a picture as possible of how you are being affected by your illness, and what may have been responsible for triggering off the problem. Possible triggers include:

• Your own susceptibility to patterns of illness (eg you may already have noticed that you develop a sore throat or swollen glands every time you feel under the weather, or that you start experiencing heartburn or indigestion when under stress).

• Any emotional trauma you may have experienced before or during the emergence of your symptoms.

• Physical stress or radical changes in your environment or eating patterns before illness set in.

- Prolonged exposure in your home or work to conditions that may be causing you worry or anxiety.

By putting this information together, your homoeopath will be able to analyse the case, assessing what homoeopathic prescription will fit your individual symptom picture most snugly. By achieving this match a process takes place in which your homoeopathic medicine acts as a catalyst, enabling your body to resolve and throw off symptoms of ill health. When this process takes place, both body and mind regain their equilibrium as they are enabled to carry out their functions smoothly and efficiently once again.

What Conditions Should Be Regarded As Appropriate For Homoeopathic Treatment?

~

Broadly speaking, there are no barriers to homoeopathic treatment, although there are certain situations that indicate that results may be limited. These include:

- Any irreversible tissue damage, such as badly distorted joints as a result of arthritis.

- Any mechanical obstacle to improvement such as a displaced vertebra.

- Situations where large and repeated doses of orthodox drugs have been taken which have masked and suppressed the original symptoms.

Even in the scenarios described above, homoeopathic treatment will still be of use as an adjunctive or supportive measure in helping to ease pain, or in helping prevent further problems.

There is no age barrier to treatment: homoeopathic patients will range from babies to the elderly. What is most important in determining the outcome of treatment is usually the strength and resilience of your individual constitution. In other words, if you have experienced a history of illness which was infrequent, short, and quickly thrown off without complications, this would suggest that you have a vigorous constitution; other people may find that an illness brings with it a host of minor complaints and that it takes weeks to throw it off. Falling ill is not the problem: it is how you recover from an illness that provides the essential clues as to what sort of constitution you possess.

43

What Conditions Should I Regard As Needing Professional Help?

It helps if you think of illness as falling into two separate categories: acute or chronic.

If we are describing an **acute** problem we can recognize it by the following features. It will:

- Have a clearly defined and limited life span with a definite beginning and end. Good examples would include the childhood infectious diseases with their characteristic incubation period, feverish stage where the characteristic symptoms become apparent (such as the rash in Chicken Pox), and the final stage when the symptoms are receding.

- Generally clear up of its own accord, given favourable conditions, within a predictable period of time. This is true, for example, of the common cold or a case of food poisoning. On the other hand, the illness can be extended if complications set in, resulting in a much longer convalescent period.

Chronic illnesses, on the other hand, demonstrate the following characteristics:

- They do not clear up of their own accord, regardless of time or favourable conditions. Good examples of chronic conditions would include Psoriasis, Irritable Bowel Syndrome, Arthritis, Migraines, and Pre-Menstrual Syndrome.

- All chronic illnesses share the tendency to repeated flare-ups which do not go anywhere towards resolving the situation.

Generally speaking, if you experience any acute illness without the complicating factor of an already present chronic condition, this will be an appropriate situation for self-help prescribing. You can acquire an adequate knowledge of first aid measures, first by attending a homoeopathic self-help class, and secondly by buying at least one of the many homoeopathic home-prescribing family guides available (see Recommended Reading).

If your problem falls into the chronic category it is always best to consult a trained homoeopathic practitioner. Managing your case may be a complicated and long drawn out process, requiring assessment at each stage by a skilled practitioner of your rate and quality of progress.

What Is The Difference Between Homoeopathy
And Orthodox Medical Treatment?

Women regularly come into contact with conventional medicine either because they need treatment themselves, or because their children are ill. Because of this familiarity, women are very conscious of the reliance of orthodox medicine on drugs or regular tests as a way of dealing with ill health.

Orthodox drugs work by opposing the symptoms produced by the body. If we take the example of indigestion, we all know that antacids will only give short-term relief. In other words, they will have a beneficial effect for a limited time, but once this has run out, we will need to repeat the dosage. The same is true of painkillers: they will dull the pain for a limited period of time, but unless the underlying problem has been dealt with, we will need to repeat the dosage once it has run out.

In contrast, a homoeopathic approach concentrates on supporting and aiding the defence mechanism possessed by our bodies. As long as we experience good health our bodies are kept in smooth running order by a system of checks and balances we call our defence mechanism or immune system. When this basic balance is disrupted through long-term physical stress or emotional trauma, we experience symptoms of ill health which communicate to us that all is not well and that we need to take action to restore the balance.

If we take an orthodox drug to knock out these symptoms it is a bit like taking a hammer to smash the warning light on our car dashboard. That light is there to warn us that something needs to be attended to: by removing the light we have not solved the problem, all we have done is put off taking action. In the meantime, our car may grind to a halt. In all probability, the car is now suffering from an even more serious problem than the one the light was warning us about.

We can regard symptoms of ill health in exactly the same way: if we attend to the problem by recognizing the factors that led up to ill health, choose a dynamic system of medicine that supports the body in its efforts to come to terms with the problem, and make modifications in our lifestyle to support this medical treatment, the results have to be more satisfying than those produced by haphazard removal of symptoms by repeated courses of drugs.

Homoeopathic theory takes this a step further by suggesting that the defence mechanism each one of us possesses will constantly try to maintain equilibrium, and when this is not possible, will throw the disturbance out to the furthest level it can reach, in an effort to keep our vital organs intact. For example, if you have been under long-term stress and develop a skin disorder such as psoriasis or eczema, your homoeopath would interpret this as your body's way of indicating that help is needed, without compromising your more vital organs such as your lungs or stomach. If homoeopathic treatment is successful, your body will have resolved the symptoms through being supported in its fight to externalize the disorder. However, if your skin disorder is suppressed through the use of a cream or ointment, it may be pushed deeper into your body because the underlying imbalance has not been addressed.

Many practitioners are familiar with cases of skin disorders which have been suppressed which lead on to more internal problems such as asthma or hay fever. This makes sense if we regard the emergence of irritation on the skin as a way of expressing symptoms on a level of the body that is least threatening to the vital organs. However, if this route is blocked, the defence mechanism has no option but to express the symptoms on internally.

You can see that embarking on homoeopathic treatment will open up a radically new perspective for you on what constitutes good and bad health. Suddenly the possibility is open to you that there are ways you can employ to support your own, positive experience of health. The excitement that comes with this discovery is enormous.

Will I Have To Make Radical Alterations In My Lifestyle?

Everyone comes to homoeopathic treatment with differing expectations and varying degrees of commitment. Some will be committed vegetarians, others may be equally enthusiastic carnivores; some patients will have a social life that leads to regular consumption of alcohol, others may find it does not feature in their life at all. The exciting aspect of homoeopathy as a therapeutic system is that it takes these factors on board as objectively as possible, assessing each case as an expression of that individual's way of living their life.

Generally speaking, it is not a good idea to make too many radical changes at the beginning of homoeopathic treatment; otherwise it may be difficult to assess what results are due to the action of homoeopathic remedies, and what are reactions to changes in lifestyle. If there are obvious factors that may be hindering results, such as frequent consumption of coffee in a chronic insomniac, clearly it would be a good idea to take care of them before anything else. Otherwise it is a bit like mopping the floor beneath an overflowing sink when all that needs to be done is to turn off the tap. There are certain substances which may interfere with the beneficial action of homoeopathic medicines: these include strong tea or coffee, peppermint flavoured sweets or toothpaste, Camphor, and certain aromatherapy oils including Rosemary and Thyme.

Don't be put off by the idea that homoeopathic treatment involves deprivation or self-punishment: as you begin to appreciate how your body can function when enjoying optimum levels of vitality, any commonsense changes in diet or lifestyle will move easily within your grasp. Successful homoeopathic treatment can give you the impetus you need to get started: once this happens extra energy is available to initiate changes or encourage commitment to an exercise plan or dietary improvement.

This shows us that it is possible to break out of a vicious circle: as overall vitality improves we have more energy to feel enthusiastic about taking exercise or cutting out foods that we know make us feel ghastly; this in turn, makes us feel even more positive because the changes we have made contribute to improved experience of well-being—and so it goes on. But in order to experience this enhanced feeling of energy and dynamism we need something to give us an initial boost to jolt us out of a cycle of eating badly and feeling exhausted: a dynamic system of medicine such as homoeopathy can provide this key to the problem.

Alternative methods of healing help us make friends with our bodies, encouraging us to learn what makes us feel good and what does the opposite. Once we have learnt to value these sensations, we can begin to make changes that seem right for us, rather than feeling that we are mechanically following advice without understanding why. The resulting freedom that comes from being in tune with our bodies is one of the most exciting and often unexpected bonuses of alternative treatment.

What if I Am Already Taking Orthodox Drugs?

Because homoeopathic medicines are working on a sub-molecular or dynamic level, they do not leave detectable traces in the tissues of the body. As a result, unforeseen chemical interactions are not likely between homoeopathic medication and orthodox drugs, because each is working from a different premise. If interaction does occur, it is normally on the level of the powerful orthodox drug cancelling out the action of the more gently acting homoeopathic remedy.

On the other hand, problems of a subtler nature can ensue if you choose to take orthodox medication side by side with your homoeopathic treatment. The problem is essentially one of suppression of symptoms as a result of the former course of treatment. This can make it very difficult for your homoeopath to establish what symptoms were originally expressive of your problem, and which current symptoms may be the result of drug-induced side-effects. Other problems include the potential disruptive effect of orthodox medication to homoeopathic treatment, as, for example, when a patient experiences a set-back after a course of antibiotics or use of steroids.

It is obvious that homoeopathic treatment is much less complicated if you come along for the initial consultation when you are not taking a course of medication. On the other hand, life is not always that straightforward, and homoeopaths are sometimes presented with cases where a patient is on a course of medication that cannot be discontinued. If this situation occurs, many practitioners will be prepared to adopt a position of compromise: putting their efforts into raising your overall vitality and constitution with a view to the orthodox drugs eventually being discontinued under the supervision of your GP as symptoms improve.

Can I Use Other Forms of Alternative Medicine If I Am Receiving Homoeopathic Treatment?

~

Broadly speaking, there is no problem in combining different forms of alternative therapy; in fact there are situations where this would be both beneficial and appropriate. A good example would be where someone suffered chronic anxiety and muscular tension which resulted in long-term insomnia. In this case it would make sense to opt for long-term homoeopathic treatment to reduce tension and anxiety, while massage would be an excellent aid to relaxation. Other examples would include any situation where there was a mechanical obstacle to improvement such as a displaced vertebra. In this situation it would make sense to choose osteopathic or chiropractic treatment to realign the spine, while homoeopathic treatment or acupuncture would make an excellent follow-up therapy.

It has been suggested by some homoeopathic practitioners that homoeopathy and acupuncture, although very similar in therapeutic terms, should not be combined at the same time because they do not work well together. Given this incompatibility, it would make sense to concentrate on one of these two therapies for a given period of time to assess results before moving on to the other.

It is generally wise to concentrate on one main therapy such as acupuncture, herbalism or homoeopathy for a reasonable length of time rather than falling into the trap of therapy-hopping. The reason for this is simple: unless you persevere with one therapy for a while it becomes very difficult for you or your practitioner to assess your progress. Once this has become clear, you are then in an excellent position to evaluate with the help and advice of your therapist what adjunctive measures would speed up your improvement. The possibilities could span the range from bodywork such as Yoga, the Alexander Technique or Feldenkrais, to mind-oriented therapies such as Counselling, Psychotherapy, or Autogenic training

Do not be misled by thinking holistic treatment must involve a multiplicity of therapeutic approaches: this is by no means the case. Very often you will find that a single therapeutic system may fulfil all your needs on the mental, emotional and physical levels. Only feel compelled to look elsewhere if you feel this satisfaction is beginning to wane.

The Homoeopathic Approach

49

Myths About Homoeopathy

With the growth of interest in complementary therapies over the past decade, many of us are likely to have heard of homoeopathy even if we do not have a clear idea of what is involved in treatment. However, misconceptions have arisen and certain assumptions are made which have led to confusion and misrepresentation of homoeopathic treatment. The following will give some idea of the most common misunderstandings:

'Homoeopathy is an ancient philosophy of medicine.'

Although it has antecedents in earlier medical ideas, the theory of homoeopathic medicine does not date back to the Middle Ages or earlier, but is a comparatively recent development in the history of medical science. Samuel Hahnemann, the physician responsible for initiating and developing the theory and practice of homoeopathic medicine, was born in Germany in 1755.

Trained as a conventional doctor, he developed the theoretical basis on which homoeopathic medicine rests as response to his dissatisfaction with the medical practices of his day. From the nineteenth century to the present day, homoeopathic practitioners have continued to see patients even though the demand for homoeopathic treatment has fluctuated according to political, economic, and other factors.

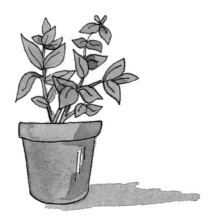

'Homoeopathy is the same as herbal medicine.'

~

This is one of the most common myths about homoeopathy, and it is easy to see why the confusion has arisen. Although plants are used in the preparation of homoeopathic medicines, they are just one of the potential ingredients. In theory a homoeopathically prepared medicine can come from any number of sources including minerals, metals, or toxic substances such as snake venom.

One of the most important differences between homoeopathy and herbalism lies in the method of preparation of the respective medicines. Herbal medicines generally involve mixtures of herbs prescribed in comparatively large quantities — typically the extract from 30g or more per day — with as many as eight or nine herbs included in the mixture. Homoeopathic medicines, on the other hand, are prepared in a highly diluted form, and at each stage of serial dilution they will undergo a process of pounding called 'succussion'. Only if both processes are carried out will the medicine be regarded as homoeo-pathically prepared. It is also common practice for homoeopathic remedies to be given as a single dose of a single substance rather than in combinations.

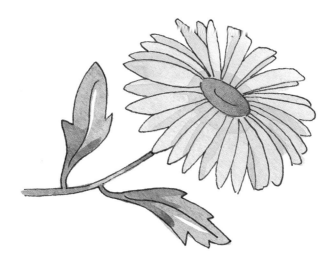

'Homoeopathy is completely safe and harmless because it is "natural".'

While homoeopathic medicines provide a safe and effective alternative to orthodox drugs, they should be treated with the respect due to any form of medical treatment which is capable of promoting rapid and powerful results. In simple cases, a member of the public who has attended homoeopathic self-help classes and who diligently uses one of the many homoeopathic first aid books can bring about exciting and rewarding results.

On the other hand, to get the maximum benefit from using homoeopathic medicines you will need to have a basic knowledge of how to select the appropriate remedy, how to administer that remedy, and most important of all, when to stop giving it. Many of the current books on the subject will give you detailed and clear advice on how to deal with these questions, and most important of all, will give clear indications on when you may be getting out of your depth and should seek professional help.

It is also essential to point out that only when the closest match is obtained between the relevant homoeopathic remedy and the symptoms of the illness will cure be forthcoming. For this reason it is absurd to talk of a homoeopathic 'flu remedy, or the homoeopathic medicine for arthritis, since there will be a wide range of differing homoeopathic remedies from which to select on the basis of the individual's own symptoms.

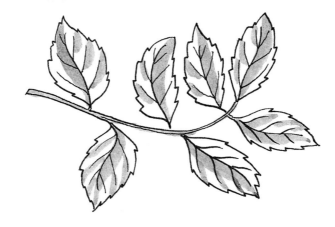

'Homoeopathy works because it is "all in the mind".'

This comment is met with very frequently by homoeopathic practitioners. Because patients who consult homoeopaths are often highly motivated and eager to see results (especially if they have come for treatment in desperation, as a last resort), the assumption is made that any cure is due to the placebo effect. In other words, because the patient feels positively inclined about the therapy, they are willing themselves to get better.

While it would be unfair and unrealistic to deny that there is always likely to be an element of placebo at work in any homoeopathic consultation, there are strong arguments which suggest this cannot explain the effectiveness of homoeopathy as a therapy. The most persuasive argument is provided by the results obtained by veterinary homoeopaths who treat, for example, herds of dairy cows for mastitis, or dogs and cats for skin diseases. There is no question that an animal cannot differentiate between being given a homoeopathic preparation or an antibiotic, and yet positive results are obtained. The same is true in the treatment of babies and young children, where favourable results are achieved on a regular basis.

The Way Forward

In this chapter I have aimed to present a positive, dynamic, and exciting approach to health care that is as much concerned with preventative measures as with treatment of illness. Most of all, this energy-enhancing approach to medicine reveals that there are systems of healing that can encourage you to make connections between physical, mental and emotional well-being; something which you may instinctively have thought possible but which you may have lacked the necessary information to put into practice. The next chapter, 'Homoeopathy in Context', will present a broader picture of how you can make many different kinds of complementary therapies part of *your* way of life.

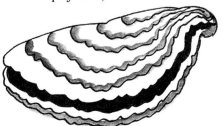

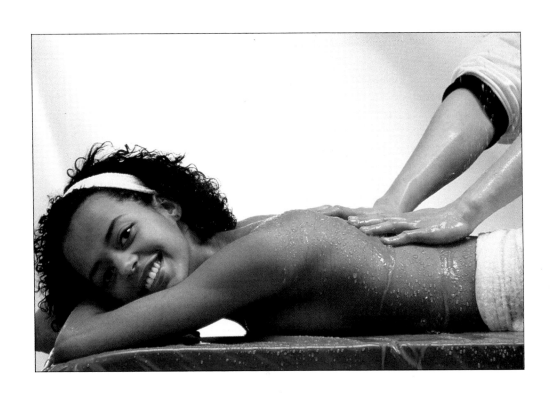

CHAPTER FOUR

Homoeopathy in Context:
The Alternatives

This chapter outlines some of the alternatives to orthodox medicine that you might consider appropriate to your needs. It is not an exhaustive account of what is available, but it will give you an introduction to some of the most popular forms of complementary medicine. It also looks at whether these therapies can be used in combination with homoeopathy.

Acupuncture

Applications
Although we may associate acupuncture primarily with analgesia, (the symptomatic suppression of pain) that is merely one small aspect of the potential therapeutic action of this ancient Chinese system of healing. When used traditionally, acupuncture may be used appropriately for a wide range of conditions including the following:

• Migraines.

• Painful or irregular periods.

• Skin problems.

• Respiratory problems such as asthma, the common cold and influenza.

• Stomach ulcers and colitis.

• Tinnitus.

The patient is seen as an individual who experiences a complex interaction between emotional, mental and physical levels of experience. Acupuncturists emphasize the importance of assisting the body to resist disease rather than just removing or suppressing symptoms.

Approach
An acupuncturist works from the basis that ill health results from an imbalance of vital energy or **chi**. When this energy flows smoothly and in harmony we experience good health on all levels. However, when this smooth passage of energy is disrupted, or the energy is deficient, symptoms begin to appear, drawing our attention to the imbalance that has developed.

In order to identify how this disorder is expressing itself, a detailed case history needs to be taken relating to the current disorder and the medical history which preceded it. Acupuncturists will also gather a large amount of information from observation of the skin texture and quality, from the appearance of the tongue with regard to shape, size, coating, colour, and moisture, and from multiple pulse readings taken from each wrist. Through analysis of the different pulses, an experienced and skilled practitioner will be able to decipher what illnesses have been suffered in the past or are active in the present, and may even be able to predict problems that lie in store for the future. In keeping with the holistic approach of Chinese medicine, acupuncturists may also give detailed advice on dietary changes that will support the body in its fight to regain equilibrium, and may also prescribe Chinese herbs to aid the body in its work.

In order to re-establish the smooth passage of vital energy once more, acupuncture needles are inserted into specific points of the body. Acupuncturists assert that a network of pathways run over the surface of the body; these are known as **meridians**. The meridians are regarded as channels through which vital energy can pass and be carried to the internal organs. By using specific points where the energy surfaces along these meridians, it is possible to manipulate the flow of vital energy in order to establish the optimum harmony between mind and body.

Acupuncture needles are very fine. Normally made from stainless steel, they vary in length from $\frac{1}{2}$ inch to over 1 inch (1.25 to 2.5cm). After use, needles will be carefully sterilized or discarded, and in the treatment of any patient who has a history of an infectious illness such as hepatitis, an isolated set of needles will be set aside for that individual and thrown away when treatment has ended. After insertion there should normally be no sensation of pain, just a small, superficial pricking sensation, a feeling of warmth or cold, a dull ache, or a sense of something moving – not necessarily where the needle is inserted. Once the needles are in place, they may be rotated to stimulate energy.

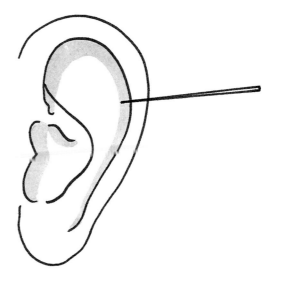

In addition, a process of **moxibustion** may be used. A small cone made of the herb *Artemesia vulgaris* is placed on the relevant acupuncture point. This is lit at its apex and allowed to burn down until a sense of warmth is experienced by the patient. Alternatively, a lit moxa stick, a little like a cigar, is held above the point. Sensations experienced during treatment may vary from temporary prickling to a comfortable, penetrating sensation of warmth. An individual session may last up to an hour and the effects of treatment may be experienced immediately or several days later.

Although it has much in common with homoeopathy as an energy-based system of healing which puts emphasis on restoring the individual to their optimum balance of good health, acupuncture should not be combined with homoeopathic treatment. Both systems work by stimulating and regenerating vital energy, but sometimes the action of one can interfere with the action of the other. In such cases, it is better to have a course of acupuncture and then resume homoeopathic treatment, or vice versa. In this way, the benefits of both can be enjoyed without the necessity of combining them.

Herbalism

Applications
The use of herbs as medicinal substances dates back to ancient Egypt and Babylonia, but the tradition has given way to a new generation of trained medical herbalists, most of whom in the UK are members of the National Institute of Medical Herbalists. Practitioners who fall into this category will generally be confident about treating most conditions unless they fall into one of the following categories:

- Life-threatening conditions that need to be referred elsewhere for emergency treatment.

- Conditions that demand manipulative measures such as osteopathy.

- Psychiatric or emotional disorders, epilepsy and neurological disorders.

- Situations where orthodox drugs are being used on a long-term basis, such as insulin. (Herbal medicines can sometimes be used to replace long-term use of orthodox drugs in a phased programme, preferably involving the patient's GP.)

- Any diseases that involve legal restrictions and restraints

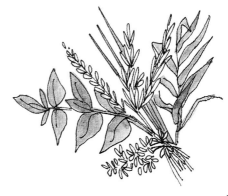

Herbal medicine is about restoring balance, and can be especially effective at supporting the action of the eliminatory organs such as the lungs, kidneys, sweat glands, bowels and the circulatory system. The digestive system in particular can be aided by supporting the cleansing and detoxifying functions of the liver.

Approach

A modern Western medical herbalist will need information regarding the lifestyle of the patient, details of her medical history, the quality of her diet, and the nature of the stresses in her life, whether emotional or physical. In addition, information will be needed about the performance of the main systems of the body including respiratory function, digestion, and emotional and nervous functions. Tests may also be conducted into the quality of the pulse, urine and blood analysis, and measurement of blood pressure, as well as other physical examinations. Some practitioners may choose to augment their practice with other diagnostic tools including iridology (the study of patterns and flecks of colour within the iris to reveal disorders within the body).

After analysing this material, treatment will begin. The main emphasis is on using herbs to encourage the body to heal itself. This can involve a combination of remedies, which may include antibacterials or anti-inflammatories to relieve symptoms, as well as relaxants, stimulants or tonics to restore balance.

Dietary advice is also likely to be given, along with recommendations for exercise or instruction in relaxation techniques to help the body return to health. The aim is to keep courses of treatment as short as possible, letting normal body functions take over the process as soon as they are able to do so. Other supportive measures that might be discussed include exercise and breathing techniques.

Herbal preparations are usually dispensed and prepared by the herbalist as mixtures which may contain a variety of different herbs. The aim is to tailor the prescription to the individual rather than to prescribe routinely for the disease condition. **Tinctures** of concentrated extracts of the relevant herbs in a water and alcohol base are most often dispensed, but herbal teas, creams, oils, ointments, capsules or tablets may also be considered appropriate.

Because herbal medicine provides a major therapeutic system in itself, there is little point in combining it with homoeopathic treatment.

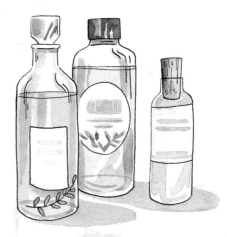

Applications

Hypnotherapy is often used in the treatment of addictions such as smoking, but its potential use is far wider than we may imagine. Conditions considered appropriate for treatment include the following:

- Anxiety, phobias and inhibitions.

- Depression.

- Insomnia.

- Amnesia.

- Stress.

- Migraine.

- Allergies.

- Digestive problems.

- Pain control.

- Asthma.

- Period problems.

- Stomach ulcers.

- Psoriasis and eczema.

Hypnotherapy is known to be effective for pain relief, particularly in childbirth, surgery or dental work. If the therapist is working with a patient who has suffered chronic pain, it is desirable that the symptom of pain be recognized not just as a physical complaint but also as a possible indication of deeper, psychological disturbance. In this situation it will be necessary to support the patient in working through traumatic emotions of anxiety, anger, guilt or despair as these rise to the surface.

Approach

If you consult a hypnotherapist, your medical history will be noted along with the details of your current disorder. Your susceptibility to hypnosis may be tested. This could be relevant if your hypnotherapist is using formal hypnotic induction and direct suggestion. However, many hypnotherapists now use indirect and naturalistic inductions, working through imagery, metaphor and other non-direct means. Susceptibility tests are not relevant in this case, since everyone can use their personal mental processes, such as imagination. A diagnostic exploration may be made while you are under hypnosis on succeeding visits. You will be taught how to achieve a state of relaxation and how to induce a state of auto-hypnosis.

Your therapist will speak in a slow, relaxing, and confident manner when inducing a hypnotic state. Images of colour, scene-setting, or repeated use of key statements can all be used to facilitate concentration. Visual concentration can also be induced by focusing on a pendulum, pencil or light. As you continue to relax the suggestion may be made that your eyes feel heavy and want to close; once this happens you are likely to be in a light trance. At this stage you will be quite aware of the proceedings and of the suggestions made by your practitioner.

In time, a hypnotherapist may take you deeper, enabling you to re-experience old, unresolved experiences that may have been buried in your subconscious mind. By bringing these to the surface with the aid of hypnotherapy it is possible to resolve inner conflicts that may be the result of forgotten childhood experiences.

Hypnotherapy can be used to advantage in combination with homoeopathic treatment, indeed, some homoeopaths may be trained in both disciplines. If a homoeopathic patient is doing well, but they stop progressing at a point where their homoeopath feels they might have hit a block of psychological origin, hypnotherapy may be of tremendous value in helping patient and therapist explore the problem area. In cases of anxiety and depression, the use of homoeopathic medicines in conjunction with hypnotherapy can do a great deal to support the patient through the trauma of panic attacks.

Osteopathy

Applications

Most patients who consult osteopaths are likely to be suffering back pain or general spinal problems. Osteopaths themselves will often see their role in a wider context, administering treatment for many different conditions, including the following:

- Sports injuries such as sprains and strains.

- Headaches.

- Migraine.

- Neurological problems.

- Digestive problems.

- Lung disorders.

Cranial osteopaths will also treat specific disorders affecting the head such as:

- Sinus problems.

- Giddiness.

- Problems in infants and children that can be referred back to birth injury.

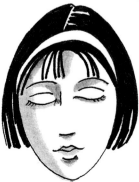

Approach

During the initial consultation a detailed history of current symptoms will be obtained, identifying their general characteristics such as when they first appeared, what appears to trigger them off and their duration. This will be put within the context of any other health problems. The patient will be observed when sitting, standing and in motion in order to identify problem areas. At this point an osteopath may require more information from further examinations including blood tests or X-rays.

Once an initial assessment has been made, treatment may consist of soft tissue treatment where muscles are massaged, or passive movement of joints by the osteopath to establish which tissues may be restricting motion. Thrusting techniques may also be used which are followed by a characteristic crunching or popping sound. This technique is usually applied to the spine or peripheral joints and can result in speedy and dramatic relief from spinal pain.

A first visit may last up to an hour, while follow-up treatments may last anything between 10 to 40 minutes depending on the nature of the problem and the approach of the osteopath.

Osteopathy can be of tremendous value as an adjunctive tool to homoeopathic treatment, especially in cases where the homoeopath attributes problems to a mechanical cause such as a misalignment of the spine or a trapped nerve. In cases of long-term trauma following accidents, osteopathy can be immensely helpful in realigning damaged joints, tendons and ligaments, while homoeopathy can do an enormous amount to aid recovery from emotional trauma.

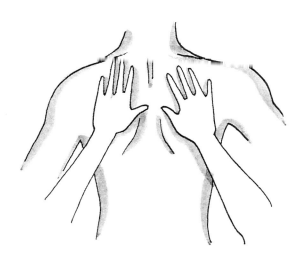

Applications

Shiatsu is a form of massage which employs acupuncture points and **meridians** (see Acupuncture, p.55). By massaging and kneading these areas, practitioners claim to stimulate and rebalance the flow of *chi* through the body, thus removing energy blocks and releasing tension. A large amount of information may be obtained from observation of the face and body of the client where areas of tension may be visible by distortion. Additional information may be gathered by the therapist from the way the client feels to touch: some areas may feel especially knotted, tense, hot or painful.

In the course of a treatment, the practitioner may make use of a number of techniques to knead, stretch, press or rub areas of the body that demand attention.

The possible application of Shiatsu as a therapy is very wide. These are some of the conditions that may benefit from treatment:

- A wide range of stress-related problems.

- Poor circulation.

- General muscular tension and lack of flexibility or stiffness.

- Asthma.

- Menstrual problems.

- Digestive problems.

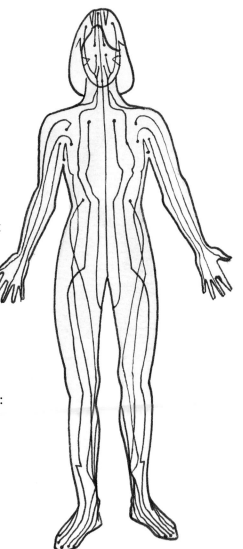

Applications

Chiropractic is a therapy that stresses the importance of correct alignment of the spine in order to maintain good health. If misalignment occurs, chiropractors claim a host of potential health problems may follow on such as digestive disorders, high blood pressure, or diabetes. The spine is brought back into correct alignment by manipulation through quick and precise movements of the practitioner. By adjusting the spine, chiropractors suggest they are restoring the optimum functioning of the nervous system, thus allowing the body to heal itself. Problems considered appropriate for treatment by Chiropractic include the following:

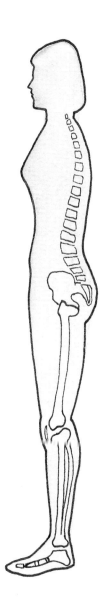

• Back pain.

• Sciatica.

• General muscle aches.

• Frozen shoulder

• Migraine and headaches.

• Rheumatic and arthritic pain.

• Slipped discs.

• Neuralgia.

• Digestive problems.

• Asthma.

Massage and Aromatherapy

Applications

Although not a complete therapeutic system in itself, massage is a very accessible and potentially highly effective supportive therapy. Most important of all, it is an excellent example of a practical 'hands on' treatment which can be received from a trained practitioner or which we can enjoy for ourselves by using basic strokes. Perhaps more than any form of adjunctive therapy, massage can put us in touch with the more instinctive, sensual side of ourselves by encouraging us to develop body awareness. Conditions that can benefit from massage and aromatherapy include the following:

• Generalized muscular tension.

• Circulatory problems.

• Low energy levels and general sensations of lethargy.

• Difficulty with relaxation.

• Headaches.

• Menstrual problems.

The benefits of massage are related to the release of endorphins from the brain, which are responsible for the same 'high' we feel after sustained, rhythmical exercise. Its exponents also claim that massage aids in bolstering the immune system, thus helping us fight illness.

When massage is combined with aromatherapy (the use of essential oils) the positive effects on mind and body are enhanced. Essential oils are understood to have a therapeutic effect by stimulating the olfactory receptors located in the nose. These convey messages to the limbic system of the brain which regulates blood pressure, memory, stress response and heart rate. As a result, aromatherapy is thought to have a positive application in conditions such as depression, hyperactivity, and anxiety. Other applications of aromatherapy oils include inhalation when added to hot water, or in herbal infusion. Always take care to check that any essential oil has been diluted in a carrier or base oil before you apply it on your skin, and avoid oral application unless supervised by a competent therapist or medical practitioner.

Massage can be of enormous help as an additional therapy for patients who are receiving homoeopathic treatment, especially if they suffer from muscular aches and pains or generalized symptoms of tension and stress. Most important of all, massage can be invaluable for patients who feel isolated, uncared for or neglected, since touch can provide the most immediate form of reassurance and communication. For those patients who are receiving homoeopathic treatment it should be borne in mind that certain aromatherapy oils should be avoided since they may interfere with the therapeutic action of homoeopathic medicines; these include Peppermint, Thyme, Camphor, Eucalyptus and Rosemary.

Applications

Reflexology is a form of foot massage which can be used for diagnostic purposes in order to identify which parts of the body may be causing problems. These organs are identified by corresponding areas of the feet feeling very tender to pressure: by working over these sensitive areas, reflexologists consider they move accumulated waste materials into the bloodstream to be eliminated from the body.

Reflexologists may also use this therapy to provide pain relief, induce relaxation and as a general tool of preventive medicine. It has been suggested that regular foot massage, in combination with a healthy diet and lifestyle has a tonic effect on the body and may be able to stimulate the body's capacity for self-healing.

In the course of a single treatment, all reflexes (pressure points) in both feet will be massaged in order to cover the body as a whole. In some cases, the hands may be used, but feet are generally chosen because they are more sensitive and provide a wider surface area for treatment.

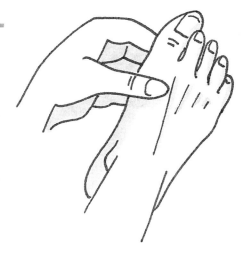

Reflexologists may be called upon to help with a wide range of conditions. These include:

• Migraine.

• Sinus trouble.

• Poor circulation.

• Symptoms of stress.

• General states of muscular tension and stiffness.

• Hormone imbalances.

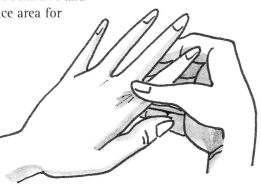

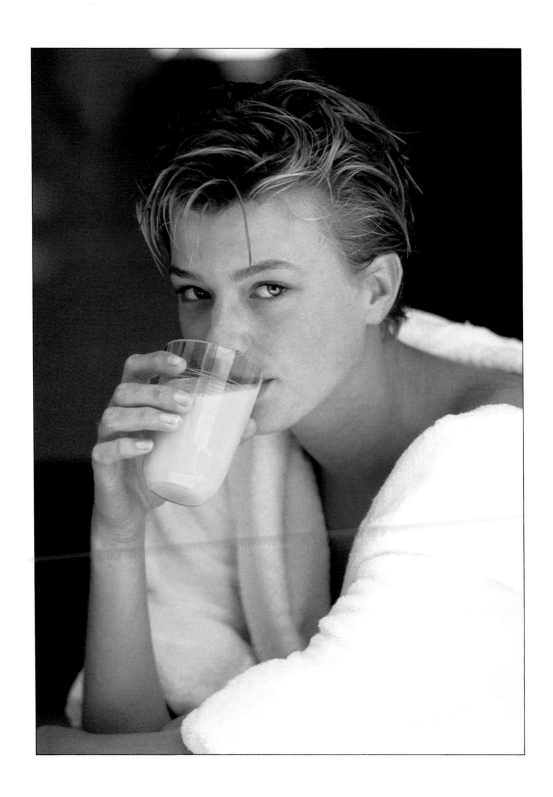

CHAPTER FIVE

Nutrition:
Maintaining the Balance

The Controversy

A basic understanding of the essential importance of good nutrition will bring you an improved sense of balance on mental, emotional, and physical levels.

Most important of all, you will discover that aiming for better eating habits need not involve great willpower, deprivation, or frustration. You *can* improve the quality of your diet and still enjoy a normal social life by going out to dinner and having friends round to eat with you

It is very difficult to see the wood for the trees these days with regard to nutrition. A multitude of different approaches exist, with each method claiming it has 'the answer'. There seems to be a new book on the latest dietary plan every week and controversy is rampant.

However, it need not be this difficult. There are a number of eating plans that have become famous during the past decade, and any sensible survey would

reveal that there are certain basic approaches that are common to each of these systems. By concentrating on the similarities we can put together an accessible and straightforward eating plan that will help us enjoy optimum health and maximum vitality.

The Importance of Good Nutrition

We literally *are* made up of what we eat: as a result, if what we consume is of very poor quality over a long period of time, we will feel energy levels flagging, be plagued by digestive problems, and look 'washed out'.

There are always exceptions to the rule: many people can cite examples of a friend or relative who smokes sixty cigarettes a day, gets only three hours sleep a night, lives on fish and chips, and still feels fine. While this may be true in the short term for that individual, there is every chance that even they will begin to show signs of strain in the long term when their energy reserves are used up. It is also important to stress that the average person will show these signs much sooner, in a generally lack-lustre state of health.

We can also reverse the picture: if the average dietary requirements are met in good supply on a daily basis for an extended period of time, the benefits are obvious and wide-ranging. Energy levels are much higher and more stable, digestion will take place without any conscious knowledge it is happening, the appearance and texture of skin and hair will be improved, and mood swings will be reduced.

This gives us just a little insight into how fundamental good nutrition is to our well-being, and how its presence or absence can affect the quality of our life as a whole.

Eating For Maximum Energy

If we want to have optimum energy levels then it is important to look to what we eat. Making sure we have enough sleep and taking regular exercise are also of great importance, but will only be able to produce limited results if our diet is poor. If we ensure that our intake of food is nutritionally sound, and we combine this with good-quality sleep and exercise, we will find that suddenly we have extra vitality and stamina to meet our goals each day.

Foods to Concentrate On

Don't be put off by any technical terms given below in the description of different food categories: where possible these are translated into everyday words so that you can have a good working grasp of the basics of nutrition.

- As much fresh fruit and vegetables as possible. These are sources of **dietary fibre**, which helps protect against heart disease. Eat raw fruit and vegetables if you can: by avoiding cooking fruit and vegetables we are less likely to destroy essential vitamins such as Vitamin C.

- Forget the idea that potatoes and wholemeal bread are bad because they are fattening: it is not the bread and the potatoes that are the health hazard, but the fat that is spread on them. Whole grains (eg brown rice, oats, rye and buckwheat), pulses and some starchy vegetables like potatoes are not only sources of essential nutrients but also supply us with **carbohydrate** to sustain energy levels.

- Low-fat sources of **protein** such as chicken and fish. These supply essential protein for building cells of the body and do not have the high saturated fat content of red meat such as beef. Although some fish, such as herrings, sardines and the mackerel family, are high in fat, it is a type of fat that is rich in healthy omega 3 fatty acids. If you are eating chicken it is important to remember that there is a high proportion of fat in the skin:

always remove it before cooking in order to allow the fat to run out during the cooking process.

- If you are using **fats and oils**, use small quantities of virgin, cold-pressed olive oil and butter. (Latest research suggests that polyunsaturated margarines may not be as good for us as was first thought, for although they certainly reduce levels of unhealthy cholesterol in the body, unfortunately they also reduce levels of the *healthy* form of cholesterol that our bodies need.) Try to make sure that your fat intake is no higher than 20 per cent of your overall food intake. Although our bodies need a proportion of fat to work efficiently, the average daily fat intake in the Western world is dangerously high and puts our health at risk.

- Drink as much filtered or mineral **water** as possible. If you buy mineral water in plastic bottles, avoid exposing them to bright sunlight, which can encourage leaching of chemicals from the plastic container into the water. If you are concerned about this possibility, choose to buy mineral water in glass bottles. Also check that sodium levels are low in mineral water if you have a problem with high blood pressure or suffer from other circulatory problems.

Remember that our bodies are made up of 70 per cent water and that we often end up taking in liquids that have a diuretic (water eliminating) effect during the day. Both tea and coffee are major diuretics. By increasing water intake the appearance and texture of the skin will be improved as toxins will be flushed more efficiently out of the body. Drinking more water is also essential for anyone with a history of cystitis or kidney problems.

- Experiment with the ranges of **fruit and herb teas** which are available. Thankfully the days are now gone when peppermint tea or dandelion coffee were the only drinks available for those who wanted to avoid ordinary tea or coffee. Increasingly imaginative and palatable blends of herb and fruit tea are on the market: they may have the tart qualities of citrus fruit, the sweetness of strawberries and cherries or the exotic taste of spices such as cinnamon. If you find a particular herb tea you are very fond of, make sure you have a break from it occasionally since you can build up a sensitivity to single herbs if they are taken frequently over an extended period of time.

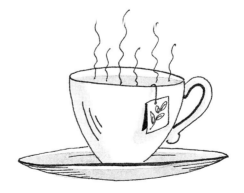

Foods to Avoid

- **Refined Carbohydrates** such as white bread, sugar or white rice. These are foods that are stripped of nutritional status and are therefore a source of 'empty calories'. In other words, we use up essential nutrients in the process of metabolism (burning up food to provide energy) which are not replaced in sufficiently high quantities by the food taken in. Take care with 'hidden' sources of refined sugar, such as fizzy drinks and tinned food. If you find it hard to give up sugar, try molasses (unrefined sugar cane extract) as a sweetener: it is palatable and contains traces of vitamins and minerals.

- Foods that are high in **saturated fat**, for example red meat such as beef or pork, full-fat milk or hard cheeses such as cheddar. Indeed, you should use all **dairy foods** sparingly and limit your consumption of eggs; although these supply excellent amounts of calcium and protein, they are also high in cholesterol, and as such should make up only a small proportion of the diet. Ways of avoiding high levels of unhealthy cholesterol include the use of soluble fibre in the diet from sources such as legumes (peas and beans), and the avoidance of a diet high in saturated fat and sugar, which in combination have a particularly harmful effect on cholesterol levels in the blood: the combination may be of more significance with regard to blood cholesterol than the actual cholesterol level in the diet.

- Overly **processed, ready-prepared foods** which are high in additives such as salt and preservatives (many of which also contain sodium). Over-consumption of sodium can lead to an imbalance between potassium and sodium in the body. While it may be necessary for convenience to make use of ready-prepared foods at busy times, make sure you don't rely entirely on them. You can also balance things out by adding fresh vegetables as a side dish or salad, and having fresh fruit as dessert. Check how many additives are included in the food: some foods will be worse than others in this respect. Remember, the fresher the food, the higher the nutritional value will be, so although some tinned foods such as tomatoes or canned fish can be useful in certain contexts, you should generally avoid foods that are tinned or dehydrated.

- **Salt** is best avoided altogether because it appears to be implicated in the development of heart disease and high blood pressure; so don't use it in cooking and remove the salt supply from the dinner table. If you include high levels of salt or preservatives in your diet you are running the risk of ingesting too much sodium. Although it is needed in small quantities to maintain body fluid balance, too much sodium in the diet can result in potassium deficiency or a tendency to high blood pressure. Using salt encourages a need for more in the diet, but once you break the habit it becomes easy to do without.

- **Coffee and tea** need to be used very sparingly, especially if you enjoy them strongly brewed. Problems associated with heavy coffee and tea consumption include palpitations, sleep disorders, and digestive problems such as nausea and indigestion.

  Be realistic about cutting down: reducing high coffee intake to zero overnight results in caffeine withdrawal, giving rise to severe headaches and jitteriness which will cause even the most strong-willed to lapse. Cut your intake of coffee down steadily and slowly to a maximum of one cup a day, and reduce tea consumption to no more than two cups a day.

- **Alcohol** is implicated in a range of health problems from liver damage to mood swings and premature ageing. Because women have a higher proportion of body fat than men, the lean tissue in a woman's body becomes flooded with alcohol sooner than a man's. This is because alcohol is not taken up by fat cells, due to their limited blood supply. Women may also notice that they are more sensitive to the adverse effect of alcohol on their emotional well-being around the time of their period. Take seriously and stick to the recommended number of units per week (14 units for women), remembering that one unit is equal to a small glass of wine, a single, small measure of spirits, or half a pint of beer. Also have at least two or three nights a week when you don't drink alcohol.

- Although cigarettes are not a food, **smoking** is a subject that falls naturally into a discussion of diet; particularly as many women refuse to give up smoking for fear of putting on weight. Vanity in this instance can be life-threatening: consumption of cigarettes is responsible for a host of health problems including increased risk of lung cancer, bronchitis, vitamin deficiency, circulatory problems such as heart disease, high blood pressure, and premature signs of ageing. The health benefits of giving up smoking are enormous, even if it requires great willpower and single-mindedness. Eating fresh, unrefined foods, taking plenty of exercise and avoiding the temptation to reach for sugary snacks will ensure that giving up smoking needn't mean putting on weight.

In order to put this information into a workable and sensible context you will find the following tables helpful. Remember that these are general guidelines, not rules that are written in stone. It is up to you to use the information as creatively as you wish. We are all individuals: what works brilliantly for one person will be impossible for another. This is especially true of our eating patterns, and a major reason why many women give up trying to improve their diet is that they just can't find an approach that suits them. The information given below sets out to inform, not to make you feel guilty about all the things you may have done wrong up until now. You will find that by using this general information you will be able

71

to enjoy the freedom of socializing without feeling guilty or unsure about what to choose from a menu.

By keeping guidelines as general as possible there is a far greater chance that the advice will be followed. This stance assumes that you do not have health problems that require special approaches to diet, e.g. diabetes or severe dietary allergic reactions such as coeliac disease. It is assumed that anyone taking on this general advice about their food consumption is in generally good health.

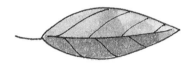

Rather than longing for the items that fall into the prohibited category, transform your approach to healthy eating by concentrating on the foods that you can eat freely. In this way, instead of seeing eating for health as a restrictive, frugal occupation, you will begin to see that many of the foods we enjoy can be part of a healthier way of eating.

The following advice will give you the broad principles of a long-term eating plan that you can adopt from now on. Of course, how you apply the advice will vary depending on changes in your lifestyle from time to time; the beauty of this approach is that it gives you the flexibility to do so.

Foods to Eat in Moderation

- If you occasionally want red meat, choose organically farmed produce.

- Butter.

- Cream.

- Cheeses such as Edam, Gouda, Brie, Camembert, Fromage frais, or some ewe's or goat cheese.

- Eggs (avoiding frying as a method of preparation).

- Puddings: have at least three nights of the week when you have fresh fruit or plain yoghurt instead.

- Coffee and tea.

- Alcohol: drink dry white wine in preference to regular consumption of spirits.

Foods to Concentrate on

- Home-made soups incorporating fresh vegetables in season, or combinations of beans that are available all year round e.g. butter beans.

- As many servings of raw or steamed fresh fruit and vegetables as possible with meals.

- White meat such as chicken or turkey. It is preferable to buy free-range, but remember that the regulations only cover the way the birds are housed, not the way they are fed: chemical chicken food or drugs may still be used in some cases, so check to make sure you are not consuming these second-hand.

- Fish of all kinds, steamed, grilled or baked, or lightly stir-fried in olive oil (not battered and/or deep-fried).

- Pasta, wholegrains, pulses and beans.

- Sauces as an accompaniment for pasta made from tomatoes, garlic and/or fresh herbs.

- Semi-skimmed milk.

- Vinaigrette made with cold-pressed olive oil and lemon juice or vinegar, instead of salad cream.

- Plain live yoghurt. Try not to add refined sugar: cinammon or honey are delicious 'extras'. Be careful when buying yoghurt-type desserts that seem to be healthy, but which when the labels are examined are revealed to contain additives, preservatives and lots of added sugar.

- As much filtered or mineral water as you find palatable: you should aim for an optimum amount of five to eight glasses daily.

- Fresh fruit drinks and cocktails that you can squeeze or liquidize for yourself.

Foods to Avoid

- Heavily processed foods, especially those that are dehydrated or tinned.

- Any food that has large quantities of salt added. Avoid cooking with salt or adding it to food.

- Foods that have a very high fat content such as pâtés, salami, or smoked meats. These may also have a high proportion of additives.

- Rich sauces containing a high proportion of cream or mayonnaise.

- Foods containing white sugar or white flour.

- Cakes and biscuits should be an occasional treat only.

- Carbonated drinks, which contain large quantities of 'hidden' sugar.

- Foods which have been subject to an array of chemical processes, or which rely on artificial sweeteners to make them palatable.

- Potato crisps and other snack foods.

- Foods that are saturated in fat such as garlic bread, unless the latter is made with olive oil.

- Chinese or Indian cuisine of the 'take away' variety or commercial versions obtained as ready-prepared dishes. Remember that there are excellent dishes included in Asian cuisine which you can prepare at home, such as stir-fried vegetables, vegetable casseroles and pulse recipes.

Methods of Cooking

There is little point in discussing foods that promote good health if we do not broaden the discussion into consideration of food preparation and cooking methods. Many foods are essentially good for us in their natural state, but can be transformed by unhealthy methods of cooking into foods we should avoid!

If we take potatoes as an example, we shall see that when they are baked in their skins they are an excellent source of carbohydrate and are even more nutritious if the skins are eaten. If we take the same ingredient and turn it into chipped potatoes, it becomes a health hazard because of the proportion of fat involved in the cooking process. The same would be true of mashed potato which is made with butter, margarine or milk. If you want to serve mashed potatoes use low-fat milk or only pepper and nutmeg.

When buying potatoes try to obtain organic varieties, otherwise the storage chemicals can be absorbed to a depth of ¼ inch (0.7 cm) beneath the skin. If non-organic potatoes are boiled in their skins, there is a risk that these chemicals can be

driven further into the flesh of the vegetable. Also make sure to peel fruit if the skin looks perfect or feels waxy: this can be an indication of chemicals on the skin. Organic fruit and vegetables may look 'imperfect', but as they have been cultivated without the use of chemicals they are far better for you than the seemingly flawless varieties in some grocers and supermarkets.

The basic guidelines given below will give you an understanding of which cooking methods preserve the nutritional status of food, and which methods compromise essential nutrients assets such as vitamins and minerals.

Healthy Food Preparation and Cooking Methods

- Raw foods! Fruit and vegetables are best eaten raw where possible, since essential vitamins are destroyed in cooking. Also remember that vitamin C content is reduced if raw food is prepared and left to stand for hours before eating. Make sure you scrub fruit and vegetable skins thoroughly.

- Steaming. This is the preferred cooking method for vegetables since it preserves a higher proportion of essential vitamins and minerals than boiling. It also helps keeps vegetables crisp and fresher-tasting. Remember that steaming is a method of cooking that can also be used for fish.

- Poaching. Useful as a method of cooking fish without adding extra fat (provided water is used rather than milk). Season the water with herbs and spices. Also a good alternative way of cooking eggs.

- Stir-frying. Excellent as a method of cooking poultry, fish, or vegetables without adding a high proportion of fat or losing the fresh texture of raw foods. Always use a monounsaturated fat such as cold-pressed olive oil rather than animal fats.

- Grilling, especially if it is done on a rack or griddle which allows fat to drain away. Do not brush additional fat on the food before grilling.

- Shallow frying or browning, either in no fat or oil at all if possible, or in a small quantity of cold-pressed olive oil. A heavy pan should be used over a steady heat. Avoid washing the pan in detergent and foods should not stick.

- Roasting. To be used as a method of cooking meat in preference to frying or other ways of cooking that involve the addition of extra fat.

Cooking Methods to Avoid

- Deep-frying. Adds a very high proportion of fat to any food, which immediately adds to its calorific value and increases the health risk.

- Adding salt in cooking. It is unnecessary to add salt to the cooking water of vegetables. Adding bicarbonate of soda to the cooking liquid of green vegetables to preserve their colour encourages the destruction of vitamins. Steaming vegetables preserves their colour naturally.

- Boiling. Not the preferred way of cooking vegetables because too high a proportion of vitamins and minerals will leach out into the cooking liquid. Boiling for an extended time also renders vegetables limp and tasteless. If you do boil vegetables make use of the cooking water in soups. Dried and soaked beans must be boiled in plenty of unsalted water. Brassicas (eg cabbages, turnips, swedes) will produce less wind in those who are susceptible if boiled in lots of water.

- Addition of fats through sauces. Always steer clear of recipes that involve the addition of a high proportion of cream or butter, usually in the form of a rich sauce. If adding a sauce as accompaniment to a main dish, choose a light tomato-based sauce which can be spiced with garlic, or purée brightly coloured vegetables such as red (bell) pepper. Remember—you do not need to lose flavour by choosing a healthier alternative.

- Fondue cookery. Avoid the hot oil method and use stock instead. Many recipes demonstrate how to use fondue pans to cook fish and poultry without oil.

Do I Need To Take Vitamin or Mineral Supplements?

Advice on whether vitamin supplements are needed or not tends to vary from those who advocate that vitamins must be added to even the healthiest diet, to those who suggest that a balanced diet will render supplementing with vitamin tablets unnecessary.

As always, the answer lies somewhere in between. Women who have a very limited diet are almost certain to be depriving themselves of certain essential nutrients, while women who smoke, drink or take the contraceptive pill may be unwittingly robbing their bodies of vitamins such as vitamin C and B complex. Exposure to toxins such as those found in cigarettes, alcohol or pollution also brings the risk of serious health problems, and certain vitamins and minerals known as antioxidants— vitamins A, beta-carotene (the vegetarian source of vitamin A), C, E and selenium— are thought to be helpful in counter-acting the detrimental effects of toxicity.

Other situations where vitamin supplements could be beneficial include exposure to infectious illness such as colds and 'flu. In the latter situation Vitamin C and Zinc can play an

important part in helping the body fight infection and help speed up recovery.

However, in the case of a woman who has a poor diet, it obviously makes more sense for her to concentrate on elevating her nutritional status through improving the food she eats each day rather than on supporting an inferior diet through supplementation. If the daily intake of food incorporates a decent proportion of fresh, raw food, protein, complex carbohydrates from grains and starches, and a small quantity of fat from dairy produce and oils such as olive oil, this should make vitamin and mineral supplementing unnecessary.

If a vitamin or mineral deficiency is known to exist it obviously makes sense to approach the problem from a dietary perspective first, and if extra help is needed, to also consider supplementing in tablet form. You need to make sure that a deficiency does exist, especially in the case of minerals, since indiscriminate use of high quantities of a single mineral can result in imbalances involving other minerals. A good example would be the administration of Zinc without establishing that a deficiency existed, since this would result in disruption of the balance between Copper and Zinc, to the detriment of the former. For this reason the fashion for megadosage of vitamin and mineral supplements should be regarded with caution.

Iron deficiency can be a problem in women because of blood loss during menstruation; women need twice as much iron as men. Pregnancy and slimming diets can also result in iron deficiency. If women have difficulty including iron-rich foods in their diet, they may consider supplementing with iron tablets. However, supplementation can cause constipation, and it is *always* best to ascertain whether an iron deficiency does in fact exist by performing a blood test. Good sources of iron in food include fish, meat, grains, fruit, nuts, vegetables and egg yolks. Vitamin C can assist in the absorption of iron, while strong tea and coffee or an excess of zinc can impede it.

The Important Difference Between Water-Soluble and Fat-Soluble Vitamins

It should also be borne in mind that there are two distinct categories of vitamins: those which can be stored by the body, and those that cannot. The former are called fat-soluble vitamins and include vitamins A, D, E and K; the vitamins that fall into the second category are called water-soluble vitamins and include vitamins C and B complex.

This information is vital to any discussion of the potential hazards of taking large doses of vitamins. If the vitamin in question is water soluble, as in the case of vitamin C, it will not be stored by the body but will be eliminated in the urine. Clearly, in this situation the chances of a toxic build-up are remote and it is generally not considered to be hazardous to take quite large doses of vitamin C for a short period of time. However, long-term use of high doses of vitamin C has been implicated in the possible development of kidney stones; so the best way of increasing your intake of vitamin C on a long-term basis would seem to be to increase consumption of vitamin C-rich foods, such as oranges, lemons, grapefruits, blackcurrants, broccoli and parsley.

With fat-soluble vitamins we are faced with a different situation, because the body will store excess quantities ingested rather than eliminating them. Clearly, care needs to be taken here lest a toxic build-up take place, as in the cases of vitamin A poisoning reported in the press. This is yet another reason for obtaining basic vitamins and minerals from foods in the diet rather than taking supplements. It is possible to eat enormous quantities of carrots and carrot juice and eventually reach the point of toxicity, but you would need to be very single-minded to do so. On the other hand, it is much easier to exceed your daily recommended intake of vitamin A by taking an excess of capsules or tablets.

Should I Eliminate Butter From My Diet?

Many people are confused these days by the apparently contradictory advice that is being given on the subject of the most preferable source of dietary fat. Nutritionists do agree on the need to cut fat in the diet down to a maximum of 20 to 25 per cent of the overall dietary intake. Keeping the general proportion of fat low, regardless of what source it comes from, appears to reduce the risk of developing heart and circulatory disorders, or cancers of the breast and colon. Because fats are also a concentrated source of calories, restricting the overall consumption of fatty foods will also assist in weight loss, especially if this is combined with a reduction in sugar intake.

Because a link was discovered between raised blood cholesterol and tendencies to heart disease and circulatory disorders such as atherosclerosis, fats which contained high levels of cholesterol were seen as fats to be avoided at all costs. Foods that contain saturated fats include hard cheeses, butter, full-fat milk, red meat, coconut oil, palm oil, chocolate and pork. As a direct response to the fear about inclusion of cholesterol-producing fats in the diet, alternative forms of fat, categorized as polyunsaturated, became fashionable: these include sunflower and safflower oils and margarines. But, as the answer to the next question reveals, this was not the end of the story.

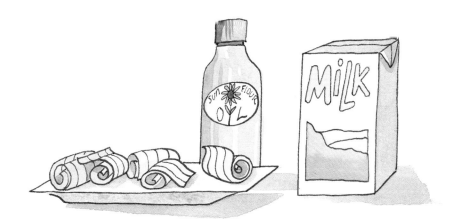

How Safe Are Polyunsaturates?

Unfortunately, many people responded to the cholesterol scare by substituting large quantities of polyunsaturated fat for their previous consumption of large quantities of saturates. It took only a short period of time for the health hazards implicit in too high a consumption of polyunsaturates to become clear; these included a potentially increased risk of developing cancer. So while polyunsaturates seemed at first to have provided the solution to the cholesterol problem, they created a different problem of their own. This concerns the presence of substances called 'free radicals', which are very unstable molecules produced when polyunsaturated fats are heated to high temperatures. When this instability occurs, mutation of these substances takes place which can render them carcinogenic. It is for this reason that repeated heating and cooling of polyunsaturated oils is a practice to be avoided, and that fats such as margarine, which are solid at room temperature, should not be heated for frying. One way of helping to counteract the effects of free radicals is to increase consumption of antioxidants in the diet: these include beta carotene, vitamin E, vitamin C and selenium (see also p.**77**).

From this perspective it is clear that the solution to the problem does not lie in substituting large quantities of polyunsaturates for saturated fat, but in reducing the overall amount of fat in the diet, whether it comes from a saturated or polyunsaturated source. If you like butter, therefore, feel free to go on eating it—but make sure you eat half the usual amount. It is also worth mentioning that cold-pressed, virgin olive oil appears to have positive qualities which protect the circulatory system, making it the preferable oil for cooking or making salad dressing. Other oils which have a beneficial effect on the heart and circulation include fish oils.

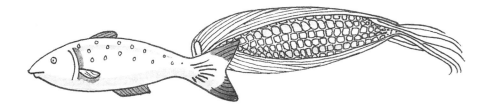

Is a Slimming Regime Necessarily a Healthy Diet?

Just as the mood of the 1990s demands a new approach to exercise which is more in keeping with a holistic perspective on health, a similar revolution is taking place with regard to nutrition. The short-cut, faddy diets of the 1960s, 70s and 80s are no longer appealing to those women who want to be at an optimum weight and also preserve maximum good health. If the message of the 1990s is about achieving and maintaining the balance between mind and body, good nutrition plays an essential role in promoting this sense of harmony.

The good news is that it is becoming obvious that an eating plan that is nutritionally sound according to the principles of good eating in the 1990s will also help us shed extra pounds. There are, of course, issues raised by the whole question of the desirability of weight loss programmes and diets for women, concerning lack of self-esteem or dissatisfaction with body image. These are issues that will be considered separately at the end of this chapter.

There is general agreement that if the dietary intake consists of foods that are low in fat, salt, refined foods, sugar in all forms (especially including 'hidden' sugar in sweetened foods and soft drinks), and alcohol, and high in fibre, unrefined foods, fresh fruit, vegetables, with moderate proportions of fish or poultry, this will give the basis for a generally sound diet. Fat and sugar are concentrated sources of calories (which is especially true of foods that combine fat and sugar together in their preparation, such as biscuits and cakes), but they provide very high numbers of calories without satisfying hunger, leaving us feeling ready for more very quickly. In addition, they are foods which are nutritionally deficient, using energy for digestion without replacing essential nutritional building blocks like vitamins and minerals. If intake of these foods is cut down drastically and more nutritionally sound foods are substituted, cravings are likely to subside.

It would be misleading, therefore, to suggest that weight loss is dependent on restriction of calorific intake alone, for the *type* of foods we eat is as important as the numbers of calories they contain. This is a controversial issue, with many nutritional experts suggesting that calorie counting is an old-fashioned and ineffective method of dieting which does not achieve sustained weight loss. It does, however, make sense to concentrate on eating foods that happen to be health promoting and low in calories at the same time, while keeping to a minimum those that are nutritionally deficient and high in calories.

Why Am I Unable To Lose Weight Even Though I Am Always Dieting?

~

We are all familiar with the syndrome of skipping from one wonder diet to the next. For many of us, following diet sheets and calorie charts is an integral part of being a woman—yet much of the information in 'traditional', calorie-restricting diet plans is both misleading and incorrect. How many women still believe that bread is to be cut out because it is fattening, or that fatty foods like cheese or meat are fine because they are proteins and therefore slimming? Today's dietary advice is quite different: fats and sugars are to be avoided, and complex carbohydrates such as wholemeal bread are fine provided they are not covered in fatty spreads.

Many women are starving themselves on a strictly controlled calorie-counted diet without realizing that the pattern of *how* we eat is just as important as *what* we eat. Writers such as Geoffrey Cannon and Susan Kano have identified that depriving the body of regular meals, and cutting down calorific intake drastically for an extended period of time tricks the body into conserving energy as a way of surviving. When this happens our metabolism will slow down (an efficient and fast metabolism is the biggest aid to weight loss), and it becomes impossible to keep on losing weight at the same rate as at the beginning of a calorie-controlled diet. Worse still, after

abandoning the dietary restrictions, the body will gain weight faster than before.

The reason for this is simple: when weight loss takes place both fat and protein are broken down, but when weight is replaced it is mostly made up of fat. For this reason, many women find themselves in the unhappy situation of yo-yo dieting from one wonder eating plan to the next, losing a little weight initially but always putting it back rapidly and feeling more demoralized each time. If you add to the equation the fact that oscillating between rapid weight loss and weight gain results in a loss of muscle tone, stretch marks and cellulite, the picture becomes even gloomier.

The answer to the problem lies in working from an alternative perspective and finding ways in which metabolism can be speeded up. One of the acknowledged ways of achieving this is through exercise, which is known to speed up basal metabolism, provided it is maintained on a regular basis. By approaching the situation from this angle, it becomes possible to eat regular, nutritionally sound meals, and still achieve and maintain our optimum weight. Also remember that it is better to eat small meals at regular intervals rather than going for hours without eating and then having an enormous meal.

Why Am I Always Exhausted Even Though I Have Plenty of Sugar and Coffee To Keep Me Going?

~

When we feel under pressure, the common reaction is to increase consumption of tea, coffee, and sugar (usually in the form of chocolate) as a way of keeping energy levels up and stimulating and maintaining alertness. While these substances will give a short-term boost of energy, there are severe problems involved in relying on them in the long term.

The first of these problems is connected to the fact that sugar and caffeine are addictive and the body demands progressively higher and stronger doses of these stimulants in order to maintain the 'buzz' or 'kick' of energy that they give. This is why it is very easy to find that we have built slowly but gradually up to a consumption of eight or nine mugs of coffee or tea a day. By the time things have reached this stage, the chances are that we probably experience unexplained jittery feelings and palpitations, and insomnia may have become an added problem.

If this is compounded by a regular intake of chocolate and by smoking, energy levels have usually reached an all-time low, and the thought of giving up our reliance on coffee and sugar has become impossible or too horrific to contemplate.

The reason for this vicious circle which ends in exhausted energy levels is very simple: stressful situations push our adrenal glands into action. If this state of arousal continues, and more and more stimulants are taken on a regular basis, our bodies are constantly relying on rushes of adrenalin to keep going. Within a relatively short period of time, the adrenal glands are over-worked and a sense of nervous exhaustion is the result, leaving us feeling like a clock whose spring is winding down.

Other problems related to relying on sugar and coffee for boosts of energy involve the action of these substances on our blood sugar levels. When these levels are stable we feel energetic and clear headed; on the other hand, when blood sugar levels are uniformly low or fluctuating wildly, we feel dizzy, sick and muzzy-headed. When we initially take sugary foods our bloodstreams are flooded with sugar and we feel a rush of energy. The body, however, responds to this influx of sugar by attempting to bring blood sugar levels down through insulin production. This works very efficiently, but has the effect of lowering blood sugar to a point where we feel more exhausted than before we took the sweet food or drink. Because most of us do not understand this mechanism, the mistaken response to the renewed exhaustion is to take more sugar in an effort to gain more energy, and so we remain caught in the vicious circle.

If this continues, infections will occur more frequently as our immune systems are compromised, digestive problems may arise from the irritant qualities of tea and coffee on the digestive system, and sleep patterns may go haywire. The way to break the cycle is simple once you have identified that the problem exists. It involves increasing water intake dramatically to help flush out toxins from the body, temporarily taking a Vitamin C supplement to help the body fight infection, making sure you have at least four helpings a day of fresh, raw food,

and choosing a low-fat diet that is easier on your overworked liver.

As far as reducing tea, coffee and chocolate are concerned, take care not to do things too abruptly, especially with regard to coffee. Caffeine withdrawal headaches can resemble migraines and if they make you feel so ill you will be disinclined to try cutting out coffee again. You need to reduce coffee intake *gradually*, replacing it with an alternative hot drink. If you choose to drink decaffeinated coffee, make sure the caffeine has been removed by a water filtering process rather than through the use of solvents which may be carcinogenic.

What Are The Arguments For And Against Being A Vegetarian?

The days are gone when vegetarianism conjured up images of nut cutlets and open-toed sandals: vegetarianism, like ecology, has become an issue which is pressing and relevant to the world we live in today. With the BSE and salmonella scares, the problems associated with meat and poultry farming became front page news. If we add to this the growing concern about the use of antibiotics in order to stimulate growth in farm animals, and the practice of subjecting animals to doses of hormones, the picture gets even grimmer.

Other questions surrounding the issue of meat consumption concern the role of red meat in raising blood cholesterol, and the tendency of red meat to ferment in the gut during the extended digestive process needed to break down the nutrients for utilization by the body. These two factors have led to the suggestion that a high red meat consumption may be implicated in two killer diseases of our age: coronary heart disease and bowel cancer.

Adopting a vegetarian diet needs planning and careful thought because it is necessary to work out where essential protein in the diet will come from. This need not be a difficult process provided beans and pulses are combined with whole grains to form a complete protein. If you consider the three food groupings of pulses, cereals, and nuts and seeds, make sure you combine any two of these groups in order to obtain a biologically complete protein. Concern about vegetarians lacking protein in their diet is exaggerated, since with a basic knowledge of nutrition it is easy to ensure that good sources of protein are included. Problems should only occur where being vegetarian is interpreted as leaving out meat and fish within the context of an already careless or substandard food intake.

It is important, however, to appreciate that mass-produced vegetables are also contaminated through the use of pesticides, and that this is a matter that vegetarians must take into account. Many vegetarians will deal with this problem by buying organically grown produce; others will make sure that they peel or scrub vegetables thoroughly before eating.

If we look at the practicalities of the situation, there are a number of reasons why adopting vegetarianism seems very difficult for many people—and the idea of becoming a vegan, which would mean excluding all animal products including dairy produce and eggs, may seem out of the question. Some will not have a lifestyle that can accommodate the restrictions, especially if they need to travel or eat out a great deal; others will just feel that they do not want to give up eating meat or fish dishes occasionally because they find them pleasurable.

For those who feel they cannot or do not want to take the step of eliminating meat from their diets, there are certain practical guidelines they can follow to improve their diet;

- Make sure you do not eat meats such as beef or pork several days running: having long gaps in between eating meat gives your digestive system a chance to recover.

- Try to locate sources of organically farmed red meat or, if this is unavailable, seek out 'conservation grade' meat farmed on conventional lines but with medicines only administered to animals on an individual (rather than herd) basis.

- If you do not want to cut out animal products, choose free-range chicken or fish. The protein in poultry or fish is more readily accessible and less stressful for the digestive system than that in red meat. If you are buying fish, try to avoid farmed salmon or trout, since these are exposed to chemicals and fungicides and experience living conditions as polluted and overcrowded as those experienced by battery hens.

- Be aware that eating large quantities of cheese instead of meat is not necessarily an improvement with regard to your health. Hard cheeses are one of the main sources of saturated fat, and should be eaten in sensible quantities by those watching their cholesterol levels.

- Even if you can't find organically grown vegetables and fruit, make sure that you still have between four to six portions daily. Remember that fruit juice can count as one portion and that freshly squeezed juice provides the most nutrients. It is better to have fresh food from a non-organic source rather than avoiding it altogether.

- Variety is an integral part of healthy eating and this is as true for vegetarians as it is for those who eat meat. Relying on a diet of chips, beans and white bread is unlikely to be an improvement on a daily

intake of hamburgers and milkshakes; just cutting out animal products does not necessarily lead to a healthy diet! The variety in taste, colour and texture found in whole grains, pulses, and fresh fruit and vegetables should make a vegetarian diet delicious and delightful to look at. Always try to vary what you eat, including as much fresh food as possible.

- Above all, remember that it is essential to keep a flexible attitude towards your eating patterns. Once dietary approaches become too rigid it is easy to lose sight of the fact that we do not just eat in order to fuel our bodies: we also eat in order to experience pleasure and the conviviality of sharing with others. If we lose this aspect of the eating experience we are losing an essential feature of our lives: loss of this vital element should not have any part in a holistic experience of living. However you choose to eat, remember that feeling relaxed is vital to a healthy digestion; feeling tense or guilty is one of the greatest impediments to the process.

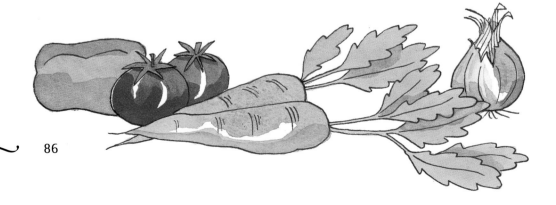

What About Eating Disorders Like Anorexia And Bulimia?

In any discussion of healthy eating and a balanced approach to food, it is vital to consider the issue of eating disorders such as anorexia nervosa. In the 1970s and 80s the medical profession was faced with a growing problem of treating young women who were literally starving themselves to death. During the mid- and late 1960s, advertising and the media generally promoted the fashionable image of the androgynous young woman who seemed to be in a perpetual state of pre-pubescent slenderness. Rounded curves of breasts and hips were seen as undesirable, and many young women who were not slim by nature starved themselves into as close an approxima-tion as possible of the desired shape.

Sadly, for many of these women the 'ideal' weight was elusive: every time they reached a target weight it was not enough, for the target became lower and lower. These movable goalposts are still dictating the fashionable shape today. The statement of the Duchess of Windsor that it is never possible to be too rich or too thin rings painfully true for many women. For women suffering anorexia the ideal can never be reached because the preoccupation with weight masks a deeper dissatisfaction and insecurity which remains unresolved.

As we moved through the 1980s bulimia came to the attention of the media as a disorder that involved the vacillation from bingeing to starvation, or the reliance on the use of laxatives or vomiting to eliminate food that had been eaten. While the specific ways employed by the woman suffering from bulimia to control her weight would differ from the patterns observable in an anorexia sufferer, certain characteristics have been identified as being shared by the majority of women suffering from eating disorders. These include:

• Low sense of self-esteem.

• Fear of losing control.

• Competitiveness.

• Preoccupation with eating and food preparation.

• Distorted body image.

• Possible addiction to exercise.

• Depression, loneliness and despair.

• Constant desire to be thinner.

As we can see, many of these characteristics are also applicable to those who are addicted to exercise, and indeed, many women come to exercise addiction by way of wanting to control their weight. Susan Kano, Marilyn Lawrence, Susie Orbach and Naomi Wolf are just a few of the writers who have explored the issues surrounding eating disorders and women. Factors which are seen as playing a part include the constant portrayal of slender, desirable women in the media, the need for women to seek assurance that they are worthy of notice through their appearance, and desire of approval from a society that values and admires those who are thin.

There are obviously other factors at work here, such as the illusion of control that dieting brings. For those women who may feel uncomfortable with maturity it is possible to arrest menstruation if body fat is reduced sufficiently, thus creating the illusion of reawakening a pre-pubescent state. If other aspects of life are unsatisfactory, it is very easy to fall for the illusion that if only one were thinner other things would fall into place. Of course, this never happens, which is part of the reason why the perfect weight seems so elusive.

Making peace with food only comes through making peace with one's body: once that happens, food ceases to involve all of the fraught, guilt-ridden emotions that surround eating disorders. For this to happen attitudes to women also need to change so that they are not led to evaluate their achievements and attributes on the level of appearance alone.

This brings us back to the concept of balance, which is at the heart of any discussion of holism: it is only in the absence of this harmony between mind and body that eating disorders can flourish.

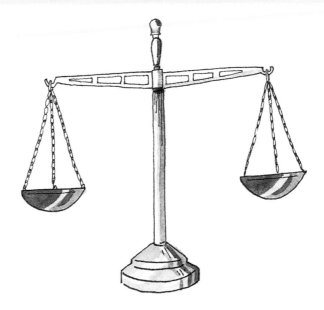

Some Popular Dietary Approaches

You will find listed below a survey of some well-known eating plans. The diets that have been included have been chosen for their variety and prominence, but this is no way intended to be an exhaustive list. This section will give you a basic idea of what is involved in each system without giving a personal endorsement of any one method.

Food Combining: The Hay Diet

Advocates of food combining argue that a sound approach to nutrition is one of the basic ways of ensuring good health. If we take this as fact, the reverse is also equally true: that a poor or badly balanced diet can also be a major factor in causing and maintaining poor health with its multiplicity of distressing symptoms, from digestive problems to painful joints.

The Hay Diet works from the premise that symptoms of disease stem from adverse chemical conditions in the body. These conditions are the result of the manufacture and accumulation of acid by-products left in the wake of digestion and metabolism in larger quantities than the body can cope with. If this process continues, a condition of self-poisoning takes place in the body. The factors implicated in this toxic process include too high a consumption of acid-forming foods such as meat and refined carbohy-

drates; and constipation, which means that toxic waste products are not being eliminated from the body quickly enough.

The differing properties of food also lead to different methods of digestion: for example, protein requires an acid medium for digestion, while starches need an alkaline environment in order to be broken down efficiently. If proteins and starches are mixed together in the same meal, this results in an insufficient acid or alkaline medium to digest either effectively.

The basic argument of food combining, then, is that we consume too many acid-forming foods and that we confuse our digestive systems by eating the wrong combinations of foods. The following tables will give you some idea of which foods fall into the 'acid-forming' and 'alkaline-forming' categories.

Alkaline-Forming Foods

- Fresh vegetables.

- Salads.

- Fresh fruit (with the exception of plums and cranberries).

- Millet.

- Almonds, Brazil nuts, chestnuts, hazelnuts, pine kernels.

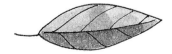

Acid-Forming Foods

• Meat.

• Poultry

• Fish.

• Shellfish.

• Eggs.

• Cheese.

• Nuts (except almonds, Brazil nuts, chestnuts, hazelnuts and pine kernels).

• Starches, grains (except millet), bread and flour.

• Sugars.

The Hay Diet proposes that a healthy, balanced way of eating involves consumption of 80 per cent alkaline-forming foods as against only 20 per cent acid-forming foods. Given that, according to the Hay way of eating, even protein meals and starch meals should include plenty of fresh fruit and vegetables, the division of daily meals ought to be as follows:

• One protein meal.

• One starch meal.

• One alkaline meal.

• It could also be two alkaline plus one protein *or* starch meal.

If you follow these recommendations and don't mix either starch foods or sugar with protein, you will be reducing your intake of acid-forming foods while at the same time allowing your digestive system to operate more efficiently.
The Hay Diet recommends cutting out refined carbohydrates, especially white sugar and white flour, which may be found in the form of cakes, biscuits, pastry and puddings and soft drinks, and cutting out refined grains like sago and tapioca. Factory-produced, instant foods that are high in additives should also be avoided.

Foods that are especially recommended include bread made from wholewheat flour; wholegrain brown rice; fresh wheatgerm and bran to increase intake of fibre; small quantities of fat, from cold-pressed sunflower seed or olive oil and from fresh, unsalted or slightly salted butter; small quantities of free-range meat, eggs and cheese; large quantities of fresh (and preferably raw) fruit and vegetables, including salads and fresh herbs, cider vinegar or lemon juice for salad dressing; and sparing use of sea salt. Cream dressings may be used with starch or protein meals. If you feel hungry between meals, *healthy* snacks such as sunflower or pumpkin seeds, fresh fruit or dried fruit not treated with chemicals are recommended.

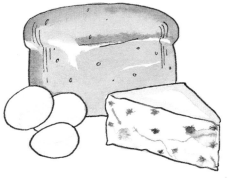

Drinks Suggestions

The following are possible options, remembering that the Hay Diet suggests that as a general rule it is best to avoid drinking with meals as it interferes with efficient absorption of nutrients from food, only drinking when thirsty.

Drinks to Consider with a Protein Meal

- Weak tea or coffee (avoid cereal substitutes, sugar and milk).

- Any herb tea.

- Fruit juice of fresh citrus fruits or berries.

With a Starch Meal

- Tea, coffee or cereal substitutes.

- Fresh tomato and raw vegetable juice, avoiding citrus fruit or berry juices.

- Grape juice.

With an Alkaline Meal

- As for a protein meal.

- Milk may be taken with a fruit breakfast.

Suggested Eating Plan For One Day

Alkaline Breakfast

Fresh fruit in season.

Live yoghurt with a teaspoon of wheatgerm.

Weak tea, herb tea, real filtered coffee from freshly ground coffee beans. Coffee may be taken with milk to buffet any harmful effects.

Starch Midday Meal

Potatoes baked in skins with butter, salad, or cooked vegetables *Or* Salad sandwich with wholewheat bread and butter.

Sweet fruit.

Bran could be included with this meal.

Protein Evening Meal

Vegetable soup (without meat stock).

Small portion of meat, fish, shellfish, chicken, eggs or cheese.

Salad of fresh, raw vegetables, cooked green/root vegetables avoiding potatoes.

Fresh fruit: choose from apples, pears, or oranges (avoid adding sugar).

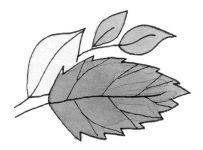

Basic Suggestions For Those Following The Hay Diet

- If eliminating sugar from the diet seems impossible, a honey syrup may be made by dissolving one tablespoon of honey in $1/4$ pint of boiled, cooled water. This may be stored in a screw-top jar.

- Try to avoid drinking with meals, or immediately before or afterwards. Drink plenty of filtered or mineral water *between* meals.

- Eat as many fresh vegetables, salads and fruit as possible.

- Treat alcohol with respect and consume only in moderation. Alcohol to be avoided includes sweet wines, sweet sherry, liqueurs, and sugar-loaded cocktails. Whiskey and gin are 'neutral', that is, they can be drunk with either protein or starch meals, but beer falls into the category of refined carbohydrate and should therefore be avoided near a protein meal. A good quality dry white wine is the recommended drink for accompanying a protein meal because it aids digestion.

- When enjoying a healthy diet, consider all the other factors that contribute to good health, such as exercise, rest, fresh air, and a positive state of mind.

The information given above is based on *Food Combining for Health: A New Look at the Hay System* by Doris Grant and Jean Joice.

The Complete F–Plan Diet

As its name suggests, the F-Plan Diet concentrates on increasing the overall intake of dietary fibre. It is put forward not only as a weight loss plan, but also as a way of enhancing the quality of the daily diet.

Possible problems implicated in too low a fibre content in the diet include:

- Propensity towards degenerative diseases such as coronary heart disease, bowel cancer, diabetes, and diverticulosis.

- Need to eat more frequently: fibrous food is more satisfying and therefore keeps hunger at bay.

- Low-fibre diets are often high in fat: problems involved with a high-fat diet include increased risk of heart disease, and excess weight. An increasing volume of evidence links high-fat diets with cancer of the breast and other common Western degenerative diseases.

The F-Plan advocates calorie-counting as a way of losing weight and maintains that a diet which is high in fibre will slow down eating habits, and be more filling. It also suggests that people who follow high-fibre diets will excrete an increased proportion of calories compared with those who eat little dietary fibre.

The recommended amount of dietary fibre on the F-Plan is set between a minimum of 35g and a maximum of 50g each day. This is roughly double the average daily consumption of fibre in the Western diet. Because fibrous matter is derived from plant sources rather than animal foods, and is not over-processed or refined, increasing dietary fibre involves a natural reduction in the following foods:

- Dairy foods such as milk, eggs, cheese and meat.

- Refined foods such as biscuits, cakes and sweets.

- White sugar.

F-Plan Dietary Rules

- Daily calorie intake should be within a range of a minimum of 850 and a maximum of 1,500 calories.

- Daily intake of fibre should be a minimum of 30g, or a maximum of 50g.

- Have half a pint of skimmed milk daily.

- Apart from milk, opt for drinks that have a low calorie content.

- Have two whole, fresh fruits daily.

- Try to obtain dietary fibre from a range of cereal, fruit and vegetable foods.

- When and how often to eat is left to the individual, provided they stay within the overall fibre and calorie allowance.

Eating Out

- Keep to low-fat dishes.

- Choose simply prepared dishes.

- Avoid hidden fats in sauces, mayonnaise, salad dressings and creamed soups.

- Avoid Chinese and Indian foods.

- Steer clear of taramasalata, pâté and cheese.

The information above is based on *The Complete F-Plan Diet* by Audrey Eyton (with kind permission of Penguin Books).

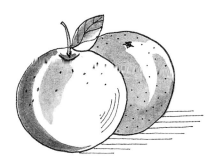

Raw Energy

Raw Energy views many of the degenerative diseases that we suffer from in the twentieth century as reactions to a state of low-level malnutrition. Although many of us may look over-fed to the point of obesity, this does not mean that we are well nourished. On the contrary, carrying excess weight can be yet another factor in predisposing us to developing at least two of the major degenerative diseases which are on the increase today: heart disease and diabetes.

Other health problems that can be attributed to a poor-quality diet include: high blood pressure, circulatory problems, arthritis, low blood sugar levels, recurrent infections, and constant sensations of lethargy and fatigue. When a poor-quality diet is combined with high stress levels, a sedentary lifestyle, and lack of exercise, it appears that one is at high risk of developing a degenerative disease. Problems with the average diet can be related to excessive use of the following items:

* Processed foods that are tinned, frozen or preserved.

* Products made from refined flour and sugar (including packaged brown bread, which may contain undesirable additives and preservatives).

* Commercially prepared foods containing artificial flavourings, stabilizers or additives to prolong shelf-life.

* Frozen fruit and vegetables and those that have been sprayed with pesticides.

* Junk fats including margarines, which contain trans-fatty acids.

* Coffee and tea.

Even if all these 'undesirables' are excluded, further problems can occur if all foods are cooked rather than eaten raw. These include alterations in food proteins, fats and fibre as well as the destruction of the 'energetic order', which can limit a food's ability to sustain health at a high level, or, in some cases, render it harmful.

Vitamins that may be lost during cooking include the water-soluble vitamins C and B. Vitamins A and E can also be lost through baking, frying, or being cooked at high temperatures.

Protein can be denatured during the cooking process, resulting in a need to eat larger quantities of protein in order to obtain a full complement of essential amino acids. If we consider that an excessive intake of protein diet can be implicated in the development of degenerative disease, it makes sense to avoid any measures that may stand in the way of utilizing dietary protein.

Fats containing essential fatty acids are damaged by being heated to high temperatures so that their chemical structure is changed from the cis form which the body needs, to trans fatty acids which it cannot use, and which can block the uptake of any cis fatty acids in the diet from other sources. Avoiding both frying at high temperatures and reheating oil already used for frying are two practical ways of rectifying this.

Suggested benefits of a diet in which 50–75 per cent of your foods are raw include:

• Increased elimination of wastes and toxins from the body.

• Restoration of optimum balance between sodium and potassium, and improved acid/alkaline balance.

• The supplying and restoration of optimal levels of nutrients for optimal cell function.

• Increased cellular ability to take up and utilize oxygen and improved micro-circulation

The arguments in favour of adopting eating patterns that rely on a large part of the diet being eaten uncooked are not new: the Swiss, Germans and Swedes have been aware of the potential healing effects of a raw diet for generations. Key figures such as Max Bircher-Benner and Max Gerson developed their ideas about the healing properties of fruit and vegetables by initially experimenting on themselves. Conducting further experiments with their patients, they discovered that food could be a basic element in curing or aggravating symptoms of illness and that positive changes in diet could deal effectively with symptoms of ill health.

The proportions suggested for a Raw Energy way of eating are 50–75 per cent raw, and the rest cooked food. More raw food should be eaten in summer and more cooked food in winter. One meal a day should consist of a large salad. The focus of one main meal a day should always be raw, and each meal should begin with raw food to avoid a syndrome of leucocytosis, an immune system reaction provoked by eating cooked food in which white blood cells rush to the intestines. If this happens every time cooked food is eaten, strain can be put on the immune system at regular intervals every day. This condition can be avoided if raw food is eaten before cooked ingredients are ingested.

Suggested cooking methods include:

• Steaming.

• Stir-frying in olive oil with a dash of soy sauce. The oil should not be heated to smoking point, and food should be cut into small pieces so that it takes less time to cook.

• Poultry, game or fish should be cooked slowly in order to retain their juices.

• Cook pulses and legumes slowly after steaming.

As well as advocating that the diet be composed of raw, fresh foods such as fruit and vegetables in season, seeds, nuts, grains and sprouts, the **Raw Energy** eating plan also puts emphasis on the

95

value of including freshly extracted vegetable and fruit juice in the diet. The suggested advantages of including freshly prepared juices are as follows:

- Being a concentrated source of nutrients, fresh juices can to be a valuable tool in both encouraging the sick body to heal, and in protecting the well body from illness.

- Helping to eliminate the accumulation of wastes and toxins from the body.

- When taken in place of solid foods they enable the digestive organs to have a much-needed rest.

- Speeding up the ability of the body to break down damaged cells.

- Assisting in bringing down high blood pressure, cholesterol, and uric acid levels in the blood.

The practicalities of eating a high raw food diet are addressed, with the following suggestions being given to those who need to eat in restaurants:

- Opt for vegetarian, Italian, or French restaurants. Salad Bars can also be a sensible choice.

- Avoid Chinese and Indian restaurants which do not have a wide range of fresh vegetables and fruit.

- Avoid items on the menu such as sauces, dressings, or buttered vegetables which include oil, cream or white flour.

- Ask for an undressed salad or add a little dressing of oil and lemon.

- Possible starters include clear soup or avocado.

- If you choose to have a glass of wine with your meal, avoid an alcoholic cocktail beforehand.

- Dessert should be fresh fruit.

- Herb tea or fruit juice should replace coffee.

Special advice is given on how to make raw meals and snacks appetizing to children, and what equipment will make preparation of raw foods quicker and easier. Possible cooked food options are listed. These include:

- Lightly grilled fish.

- Organic lamb's liver.

- Free range poultry or game.

- Fresh seafood.

- Free range eggs.

- Baked potatoes.

- Brown rice, millet or buckwheat.

- Toasted nuts and seeds.

- Soups.

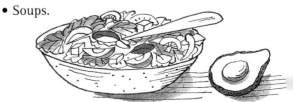

Practical advice on how to make the transition from the average diet of convenience foods to a high raw diet is given, as well as a range of recipes which include hors d'oeuvres, main salad meals, soups, dressings, dips, bread, desserts, and juices.

All of the above information has been taken from *Raw Energy* by Leslie and Susannah Kenton.

The Wright Diet

The Wright Diet was evolved as a way of eating for maximum energy and well-being. It is based on the need for the optimum balance between acid and alkaline foods in the diet. The ideal diet should include 60–75 per cent alkaline foods, but in reality, most people consume meals made up of 95 per cent acid-forming foods. Good examples of alkaline foods would include potatoes, vegetables and orange juice, bearing in mind that alkalinity can be lost through cooking water or neutralized by the acidity of frying oils.

The problems involved with eating the wrong combination of foods at the same meals are illustrated by the following example: if bread and cheese are eaten together, cheese needs an acid environment for efficient digestion, while bread requires an alkaline medium. The bread is partly broken down by the ptyalin secreted in the mouth, but by the time it reaches the stomach it mops up the stomach acid, leaving the cheese without adequate acid for digestion. If we apply

these same rules to a meal that consists of steak (protein), bread (carbohydrate), and potatoes (starch), we can see that the starch and carbohydrate will impede the digestion of the protein, making the process much more lengthy than is necessary. This will cause the meat to ferment, leading to symptoms of bloating and intestinal gas. If we add to this meal apple tart and cream (refined carbohydrate, sugar and a high proportion of fat) we can see that digestion is up against even more formidable odds.

Essential Aspects of the Wright Diet

- When eating for high energy levels, cut out biscuits and cakes: replace them with fresh nuts and seeds, whole grains, oats or pulses. If cakes are removed from the diet, it often follows that coffee and tea intake will be reduced as well.

- Try to obtain organically produced food in an effort to avoid problems involved in ingesting artificial fertilizers, pesticides and fungicides. This also cuts down on the risk of exposure to antibiotics or growth hormones administered to animals in order to increase their weight.

- Eat half your food raw to ensure high vitamin and mineral content. Foods which must be cooked include meat, eggs, and members of the bean family. Some people cannot digest muesli even if it has been soaked overnight to help break down the starches. In this situation you can try hot-soaking muesli, or making it into a porridge by quick cooking which still retains the fibre.

- Cook simply, avoiding frying because it renders oils and fats unstable.

- Cut out salt, which stimulates the adrenal glands, giving us a temporary 'lift' leading to exhaustion later.

- Keep blood sugar levels stable by eating little and often from the alkaline foods suggested above.

- Avoid foods that have been chemically processed and which contain a wide range of preservatives and flavourings.

- Use food supplements wisely.

Within the context of healthy eating according to the principles of the Wright Diet, it is suggested that food testing may be carried out to discover what foods may be causing allergic responses. (Guidelines are given for individuals to test themselves.) Foods that may be offenders include red meat and dairy products, grains and grain products, eggs, white meat, fish, nuts, fruit, sweeteners, vegetables and caffeine. Any foods that do not cause reactions may be included in the Wright Diet according to the principles given in the tables below: foods are divided into three categories.

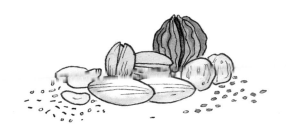

Class One Foods for High Level Health and Energy

- Fresh vegetables, ideally eaten raw.

- Unsprayed fresh fruit.

- Dried fruit, free of sulphur dioxide and mineral oil: look for organically grown.

- Honey and other natural, unrefined sweeteners such as molasses.

- Whole grains: oats, rye, barley, maize, rice and buckwheat.

- Fresh seeds and sprouted pulses.

- Fish.

- Seaweeds.

- White meat.

- Yoghurt: goat's or sheep's.

- Vegetable oils, especially cold-pressed virgin olive or sesame oil.

- Water, avoiding tap water which may be contaminated with toxic metals such as lead, copper or aluminium.

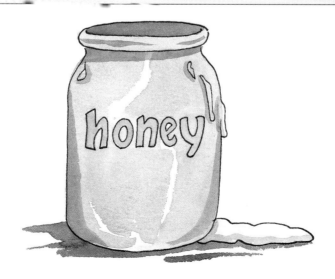

Class Two Foods which can be included in Moderation

- Cheese: low-fat varieties that are free of artificial colouring (avoiding altogether those that are processed or smoked).

- Minimum quantities of beef and lamb, choosing lean cuts and removing fat. Avoid meat that may contain residual doses of antibiotics and hormones.

- Wholewheat bread: maximum of two slices daily.

- Milk: ¼ pint daily.

- Cheese: ½ lb per week.

- Butter and margarine: 2oz of either per week.

- Eggs: should be free range and additive-free. Avoid frying as a way of preparation.

- Nuts: these should be unsalted, unroasted, fresh and whole. Avoid peanuts.

- Caffeine and caffeine-free drinks (taking note of the method of extraction: it should be a water-based method rather than a chemical method).

- Alcohol: choose organic wine and cider: avoid spirits. Be careful with organic wine and beer because of the sulphur dioxide and other chemicals which are used to sterilize bottles and equipment: some people can react adversely to these.

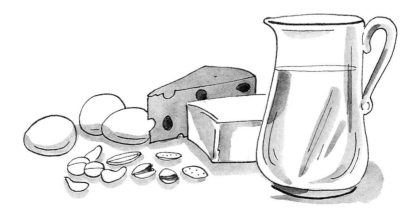

Class Three Foods which are Not Allowed on the Wright Diet

- Pork.

- Preserved and smoked meats.

- Any smoked foods.

- Cream.

- Commercially prepared frozen food.

- Refined flour products including bread, biscuits, pastry and doughnuts.

- Any food containing chemical preservatives, colourings and flavourings.

- Fried foods, or burned and browned foods.

- Instant coffee.

- Spirits.

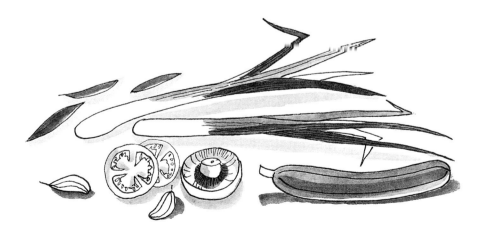

A Fast Day is incorporated into the Wright Diet for the following reasons:

- Fasting enables the body to rid itself of toxic waste which has built up from sluggish eliminative processes, or from exposure to chemicals or food additives.

- Excess weight and fluid will be shed.

- Feelings of enhanced vitality and energy can be experienced as a result of detoxification.

- Thinking processes become clearer.

- Because body cells are broken down more swiftly and replaced quickly during fasting, skin appearance will improve.

Fasting is not always desirable or appropriate: always get medical advice first, especially if you suffer from any health problems such as migraine, or if you are pregnant. For some individuals a fruit and vegetable fast may be more appropriate.

The Wright Diet also gives specific advice on weight loss, insomnia, PMS, and mood swings. All the information given above has been taken from *The Wright Diet: Your Personal Plan for Permanent Weight Loss* by Celia Wright.

The Montignac Method

The title of Michel Montignac's book *Dine Out and Lose Weight* gives a strong clue to the main preoccupation of the contents: how is it possible to eat out and still keep weight down? As well as a weight reduction plan, Montignac's approach gives basic advice on healthy eating according to the French approach to nutrition.

Calorie-counting is not advocated in this plan, since effective weight loss is seen as being intimately linked to regulating the action of the pancreas. If we keep fluctuating between low or excessively high blood sugar levels, the pancreas, which secretes insulin in order to keep blood sugar levels stable, becomes overworked and our bodies build up fat reserves. Two ways of combating this situation are:

Recognizing that refined, prepackaged foods contain astronomical amounts of sugar, starch and preservatives.

Organizing eating patterns so that meals are eaten at regular intervals, rather than starving for long periods of time and then compensating by eating enormous amounts.

The following are seen as positive factors in the French diet:

Increased amount of dietary fibre from the substantial amount of green vegetables eaten on a regular basis.

Avoiding regular consumption of sandwiches or hamburgers.

Low refined sugar intake. French people consume almost half the quantity per head of refined sugar consumed by Americans.

More wine consumed than Americans (on the basis that people in Europe, who drink wine regularly, have a lower incidence of cardiovascular disease than Americans; Michel Montignac cites evidence suggesting that wines rich in tannin, such as red wine, contain procyanidine, which can lower blood cholesterol).

Regular pattern of eating each day, with each full meal consisting of starter, main course, and final course of dessert or cheese.

The Montignac approach favours elimination from the diet of 'bad' carbohydrates which raise blood sugar. These include the refined sugar in cakes, biscuits, pastries and pasta, and refined flour: white bread is made from bleached flour stripped of its fibre, and because more glucose is released during digestion of white bread it is therefore more fattening.

'Good' carbohydrates are those that do not raise blood sugar abruptly, such as brown rice, beans or pulses, and wholewheat bread, provided they are not combined with fat.

Fats are also divided into 'good' and 'bad' lipids: fats that raise blood cholesterol such as those found in meat, butter, preserved meats, cheese and lard are seen as pernicious. 'Good' fats include olive, rapeseed, and sunflower oils. The oils from fatty fish such as salmon, herring, sardines and mackerel are also beneficial as they guard against circulatory disorders such as thrombosis.

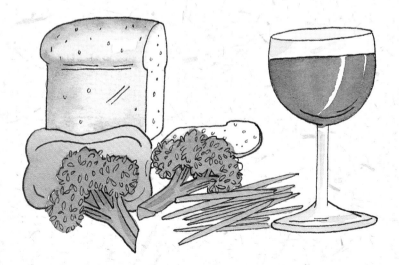

Ways of Reducing Blood Cholesterol

- Reduce consumption of saturated fat, as found in meat, butter, and whole-fat dairy products.

- Eliminate foods that raise blood sugar levels: refined flour, sugar, corn and potatoes.

- Use olive, grain and fish oils.

- Include lentils and beans in the diet.

- Eat more fish.

- Increase your consumption of fruit and vegetables.

- Ensure that you have enough Vitamin C, Vitamin A, Selenium, and Vitamin E in your diet.

- Limit your coffee intake; and avoid espresso coffee altogether.

- Eliminate soft carbonated drinks and beer.

- Stop smoking.

- Reduce salt intake.

- Drink red wine in reasonable quantities.

- Consider relaxation methods as a way of managing stress levels.

Approaches to Healthy Eating on the Montignac Method

- Never drink alcohol on an empty stomach.

- Always eat fruit on its own, and never combine it with fats, proteins, or other carbohydrates. If fruit is combined with fatty foods, it will remain blocked in the stomach instead of travelling to the intestine where digestion normally occurs. As a result, the fruit stays in the stomach for too long, where it ferments and produces alcohol. Eat fruit on an empty stomach, late at night, or mid-afternoon: at least 3 hours after lunch or 1 hour before dinner.

- Drink in between meals when thirsty.

- Combine foods with care: do not mix carbohydrates with fat, keep to separate protein or carbohydrate meals.

- Avoid sugar in all forms and the following: refined foods such as white bread, rice and pasta; starchy foods with a high glycaemic index such as potatoes; beer.

Dietary Balance in The Montignac Method

- Select poultry instead of red meat.

- Include fish in the diet.

- Ensure daily consumption of dairy products as a source of calcium.

• Select the kind of carbohydrates that prevent blood sugar levels from peaking; eliminate refined carbohydrates.

• Ensure the overall intake of fibre from wholewheat bread and cereal is high.

Detailed advice is given on how to select from menus with care, how to avoid drinking alcohol without making a fuss, and how to keep following the method once the initial weight loss phase is over.

The information given above has been taken from *Dine Out and Lose Weight: The French Way to Culinary 'Savoir Vivre'* and *Eat Yourself Slim* by Michel Montignac.

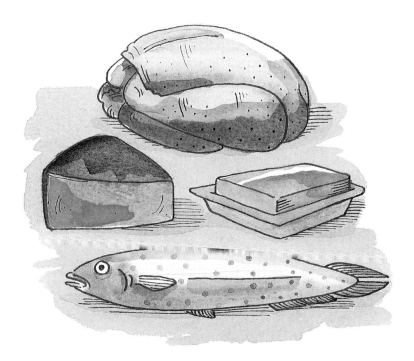

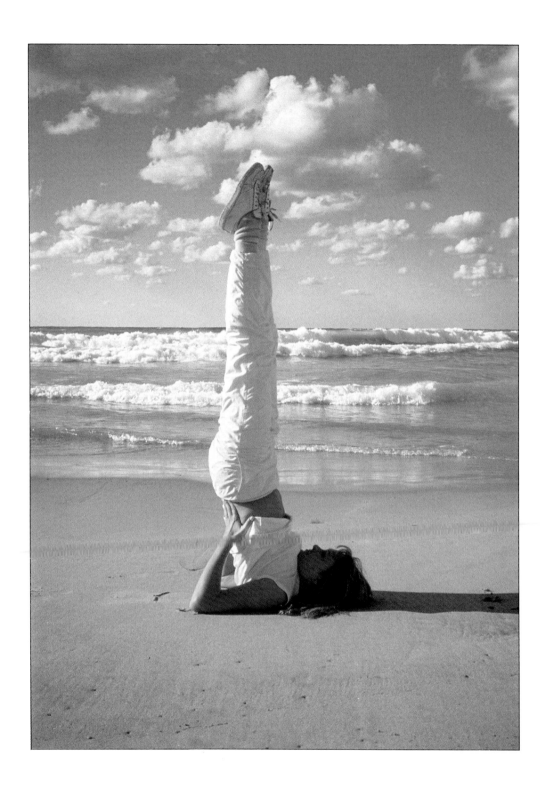

CHAPTER SIX

Body Work and Relaxation

Why Exercise?

By now we all know most of the reasons why exercise is good for us. However, it is time for a new approach to the subject which brings it up to date. The new model of exercise which is emerging in the 1990s is one which emphasizes balance, harmony, and well-being of both mind and body.

Most important of all, exercise is moving beyond the confines of the exercise class into the home. The advent of a variety of well-produced and informative home video tapes means that instead of exercise being something that is separate from the rest of daily life, it is increasingly being seen as an *integral part of life*. This new, integrated model of physical activity is vital to those women who may have felt that the atmosphere of a high-powered class was not for them. The revelation that exercise need not be competitive or a chore and that even walking is an excellent aerobic activity changes our perception of what is involved in fitness, and most important of all, of our own capabilities.

So exercise need not be a treadmill of duty and ruthless application; we can get fit doing the things that we enjoy. Many classes now on offer bring this philosophy to life by creating an atmosphere which is non-competitive and relaxed, putting the emphasis on personal tuition rather than packing in as many people as possible.

Stress and Exercise

In the pursuit of a dynamic state of health, exercise plays a vital role. Through it we can get in touch with our bodies; something so often neglected in a busy lifestyle. We can only ignore our bodies for a limited period of time; once we go beyond this limit early signs of burn-out emerge, which will continue to get more severe until action is taken.

Beyond the physiological considerations, it is increasingly clear that physical exercise plays an essential role in stress-reduction. While some of us may not be interested in the condition of our bodies, if we care about our mental performance and emotional well-being, exercise is something that must be taken seriously as a way of increasing our potential. Even if we look to our diet, sleep adequately and enjoy our work and social life, therefore, we are still limiting our potential if we ignore the importance of exercise.

A New Model of Exercise for the 1990s

The 1980s were the decade of the fitness boom: terms like 'workout', 'going for the burn' and 'pumping iron' were part and parcel of the competitive atmosphere of the decade. While the high profile given to fitness and exercise classes at this time had its positive elements, it was a period when achieving the perfect body was the highest priority, often at the expense of other considerations.

Exercise classes in particular were very competitive and often unsympathetic to the needs of the unfit individual who needed to take things at a slower pace. At this time 'going for the burn' was far more important than listening to your body, and many women ended up thinking that exercise must be either painful or exhausting.

It is clear that attitudes are now changing, and that we need a fresh approach to exercise that mirrors the 1990s

concern with a more holistic way of life. Exercise that concentrates only on the body is no longer acceptable; we need to experience a full range of activities that enhance feelings of well-being and vitality.

Getting the Balance Right

Because the 1980s convinced us that exercise is something done separately from the rest of our daily routine, preferably neatly compartmentalized in a class, many women have been led to feel that they just don't have the time or necessary commitment to getting themselves fit.

It is my hope that, in reading this chapter, you may begin to see that there is a whole new perspective on exercise, and that all you need to do is to take a fresh look. Once your perception of exercise changes, you will gradually see yourself transformed from someone who has always thought of exercise as not being for them, into someone who starts to take pleasure in their body as its strength and fitness increase.

These changes take place by making quite small adjustments, incorporating enjoyable activities into your life which encourage you to experience increased body awareness.

Freedom From Boundaries

The range of potential activities open to us is amazingly wide and we can *all* discover ways of exercising that will be appropriate to us as individuals. This emphasis on individual wholeness is very important, as it is part and parcel of the shift towards holistic thinking in this decade. People are waking up to the fact that what is appropriate for one person will not be satisfying for another, whether this involves choices in health care, diet, or general lifestyle.

Some of us are not remotely interested in running marathon races, body building or high impact aerobic work outs, but this does not mean that we don't enjoy playing tennis, swimming, aqua aerobics, or walking. It is vital to find a way of exercising that you enjoy, since you will be involved in something that is fun and absorbing rather than just dutifully exercising for the sake of it.

It's just a question of looking beyond the forms of exercise you may have rejected before, and using your imagination to investigate possibilities that are more appealing.

A Question of Sport

The range of sporting activities open to you is very wide and can include anything from playing tennis, to badminton, swimming, skiing, volleyball, cycling, trampolining or anything else

that appeals to you. If some of these were activities that were available at school and the way you were taught put you off for life, this may be why you feel that exercise is just not an option for you. You will be surprised if you try these activities as an adult just how much fun they can be. Rediscovering the sheer enjoyment of playing sport with friends can do an enormous amount to improve your social life, increase your vitality and boost your confidence all at once.

The fact that exercise can widen your circle of friends and inject more life into leisure time is very surprising to anyone who believes that exercise must involve pounding the pavements as a solitary, ardent jogger. We all need time to ourselves in which to relax and unwind, and often may feel that we want to do some Yoga or stretching exercises alone. But at other times walking or going for a swim with a group of friends may be what feels appropriate to our mood.

Overall Benefits of Exercise

Exercise and the Immune System

There are numerous hidden benefits to regular exercise, one of the most important being the conditioning and supporting of the immune system. We are totally dependent on the efficient working of our immune systems for protection against disease. One of the integral elements of an efficient immune response is a healthy lymphatic system, which includes the lymph nodes located in the neck, groin and armpits.

Toxins and dead cells are carried by lymphatic fluid via the lymphatic vessels to the lymph nodes which filter out any impurities. Once the lymphatic fluid has been filtered, it is channelled back to the bloodstream. For this essential process to be carried out, the lymph system is dependent on the natural pressure of muscles as the body moves, or on the force of gravity. Unlike the circulatory system which has the powerful pumping action of the heart to propel the blood around the body, the lymphatic system depends on muscular contractions to keep lymph flowing.

If we take regular exercise which involves rhythmic muscular contractions, this has the beneficial effect of stimulating and supporting the eliminative, water-balancing and nourishing actions of the lymphatic system. If we consider that the lymph nodes are the origin of antibody production, the role of the lymph nodes in contributing to healthy functioning of the immune system becomes clear. Stimulating lymph activity is also invaluable in helping to deal with cellulite (the pitted, 'orange peel' skin that can develop on thighs and buttocks).

Exercise and the Mind

Most of us think of exercise making us feel good because of this being the inevitable spin off of looking better as our bodies become more slender, flexible and leaner. There is also the sensation of pleasure to be gained in a body that moves with ease, and the sense of freedom and exhilaration to be gained from running. But, beyond all of this, there is a chemical process which takes place during sustained exercise which has a direct effect on emotional well-being.

This involves the secretion of chemicals called endorphins into the bloodstream, which produce pleasure-giving sensations and enhanced feelings of well-being. Endorphins are natural painkillers which have a calming effect, and are responsible for the 'high' that follows aerobic exercise.

Blood Sugar Levels

In association with endorphin production, regular exercise is also an excellent way of reducing stress. Long periods of stressful activity result in overproduction of adrenalin, with the added consequence of unstable blood sugar levels. When stress levels are high there is a tendency to rely on 'quick fix' foods and drinks such as coffee, tea, and sugar. While these will give an initial rush of energy, this will be soon followed by a further plummeting of energy levels as the pancreas over-secretes insulin as a way of rectifying the situation. What follows is a situation where blood sugar levels are swinging from one extreme to another, leading to low energy levels, dizziness, and general feelings of being unwell.

If the stress and 'quick fix' response continues then a downward spiral is inevitable, leaving us with lower and lower energy levels. Exercise can provide the necessary release by breaking the chronic stress pattern, which is especially relevant to those who work at a desk all day. In the latter situation stress can build up in the absence of any form of physical release which could diffuse the situation.

Exercise, then, provides an excellent channel for the utilization of excess adrenalin and increases the blood supply that transports oxygen and nutrients to each cell in the body. It can either tranquillize or energize, depending on your individual needs and the combination of exercises that you choose. As the body begins to work more efficiently more energy is conserved than before—and increased fitness is the result.

Breathing Correctly

To get the maximum benefits from whatever exercise you do, learning good breathing techniques is essential. Because most of us do not have to think about how we are breathing for this basic function to take place, it is easy to overlook what is happening. By learning very simple breathing techniques we can find that it is possible to be more in tune with our bodies, and that stressful situations can immediately become less threatening.

By concentrating on our breathing technique while exercising, we will find that dizziness and lightheadedness becomes less of a problem, while breathing into a stretch can increase flexibility and encourage relaxation. Certain forms of exercise such as Yoga incorporate a central concept of breath control and regulation as a way of deepening relaxation and calming the mind.

Always be conscious of your breathing technique when exercising in order to get the maximum benefit from the physical activity you have chosen to do. This is especially true of aerobic exercise: never hold your breath when engaging in aerobic exercise, and remember that you should be able to hold a conversation with ease and without gasping if you are working at an appropriate level of activity. If you have gone beyond this point and find difficulty in catching your breath, you are likely to have entered a phase of anaerobic activity which is totally counterproductive since your body is unable to make maximum use of the oxygen you are taking in. If this occurs, always slow down until you have reached a point where you can speak without strain and try to maintain that level.

It is also important to remember that the expelling of carbon dioxide is a major agent of detoxification, as the byproducts of oxidation and energy release are removed from the body. By ensuring that we breathe out to our full capacity we are more capable of taking in and utilizing the amount of oxygen available to the body with each inspiration.

First Steps in Breathing Technique

Most of us automatically breathe from our upper chest, especially in situations which are tense and anxious. In order to facilitate relaxation and an increased sensation of tranquillity, we need to learn and develop the skill of breathing from the diaphragm.

The best way of experiencing how diaphragmatic breathing feels is to lie on the floor with your knees bent and your feet about a foot apart. Rest one hand lightly on your stomach around the level of your navel. As you breathe in, feel the breath gently filling your lungs and pushing your hand up and outwards as your abdomen also expands. When you breathe out, first feel your hand sinking back down as your abdomen flattens and your lungs expel carbon dioxide.

Don't worry if this feels strange at first: with practice it gets progressively easier and feels more natural. It takes time to unlearn an ingrained habit like breathing from the upper chest. If you feel light-headed or dizzy at first, just take a few natural breaths until you feel back to normal. Never force the breath; you need to feel as relaxed as possible and to set a pace that you feel comfortable with.

You can also try the same exercise sitting in a straight-backed chair if you feel more comfortable in this position. It often helps to visualize a balloon slowly inflating with air and extending from your lungs to your abdomen as you breathe in, and the same balloon emptying itself as you breathe out. Always make sure you breathe out fully, letting out all of the air that has been taken in. By doing so you are ensuring that you can fully utilize each new breath of air that enters your lungs.

Once you have mastered this basic technique you can use it to your advantage every time you feel anxious, tired or under stress. The more we breathe from the upper chest when we are anxious, the more panicky we are likely to feel as the ratio between oxygen and carbon dioxide in our bodies is disturbed. The more regular and relaxed our breathing becomes, the calmer we feel as the balance between oxygen and carbon dioxide is adjusted to its optimum level.

What Kind of Exercise?

With the amount of choice available these days with regard to exercise, it is easy to get paralysed into immobility and find that we end up doing nothing because we simply can't decide what to do. In order to make the choice, it is essential to do the following:

• Work within your own special needs: ask yourself, 'How fit am I already?', 'How much time can I realistically make available?', and most important of all, 'What am I likely to enjoy most, given my temperament?'

- Work within the amount of time you can make available and you will find that you still get results. This will give you the incentive to make it part of your day-to-day routine.

- Find out what the basic forms of exercise do for you, and which you feel you need to give priority. A basic outline is given below so that you can choose which form is most pressing for you.

- If you use your imagination and discover a form of physical activity you enjoy, you will be surprised how your self-image can change.

- Rediscover exercise as an adult: you will find that you can become far more fit and flexible as an adult than you were as a teenager. Discovering stores of energy you never knew you had can be the best rejuvenator possible.

- If exercise is new to you, work at a gentle, steady pace that you feel comfortable with. You don't have to do everything at once: part of the fun and excitement is watching yourself gain flexibility and stamina.

- Make sure that the programme you choose is fun and pleasurable for you: once you get bored, change to another form of exercise and you will find you have renewed enthusiasm.

It's Never Too Late

Many women lack self-esteem and have a poor self-image. For some, this leads to an inevitable vicious circle of dieting, followed by bingeing, followed by guilt which leads to more dieting. Because a woman caught in this trap is constantly feeling at war with her body, she is often left with the feeling that her body is a liability, or something that she would rather not look at. This separation between mind and body leads to feelings of resentment, conflict, and dissatisfaction which grossly undermine self-confidence.

By exercising, many women find they discover a feeling of harmony with their bodies which they have not experienced before, and most important of all, a feeling of pride in what their bodies are capable of. Once this potential is discovered, self-perception can change into something positive and dynamic, things can seem less out of control and the possibility of change becomes a reality.

How Do I Work Out Where to Start?

First of all, establish what areas of your body are making their presence felt. In good health, you should not be aware of the functioning of various bodily systems: pain or discomfort are the body's way of telling you that all is not well in that area.

1. Bring your attention to your body and notice as you are standing or sitting where you feel stiffness or tension. Walk about and mentally observe how your body feels in motion: which areas feel free and flexible, and which feel tight and uncomfortable? If a lot of areas feel tight and stiff you need to concentrate on exercises which promote **flexibility**.

2. Bend, kneel, and get up from a sitting position. How fluid were those movements? Where did you feel strain or tension? Did your joints feel stiff or crack?

   For areas that feel tense and strained you should concentrate on a combination of exercises activities that combine work on **flexibility** with **relaxation.**

3. Next time you walk at a brisk pace, or climb two or three flights of stairs how out of breath are you? Can you maintain a conversation immediately afterwards, or are you too breathless to do so with ease? Do you feel dizzy or lightheaded, or are you conscious of your heart beating very fast?

   Problems in this area would indicate that you need to improve **aerobic fitness.**

4. If you carry heavy weights such as shopping bags for an extended period of time how quickly do your arms tire? How much do your arms ache afterwards?

   Problems here would suggest the need for working on **muscular strength and endurance.**

5. As you sit at your desk at work, or relaxed in front of the television, bring your attention to your jaw: how clenched tight is it? If you are holding a pen, are you gripping it for dear life with your fingers clenched around it so that the knuckles show? How do your neck and shoulders feel? How tense is your lower back?

   Any problems here would suggest that you need to concentrate on ways of **relaxing** through specific relaxation techniques or exercise which encourages relaxation.

If you find you have problems with all of the situations outlined above, you need to select an all-round programme which helps with promoting flexibility, cardio-respiratory fitness (conditioning the heart and lungs), muscular endurance, and relaxation. This may sound a tall order, but in the tables below you will find clear indications which clarify which forms of exercise promote each area of fitness.

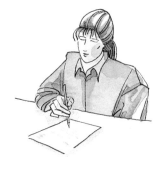

Lack of Flexibility

If you need to increase your flexibility, try one of the following:

• Stretching

• Yoga

• Pilates

• Holistix

• Medau

Do your chosen exercises every day if possible, but you can begin by setting aside 15 minutes two or three times a week. You can gradually build up to 45 minutes of exercise which you can do four or five times a week. Leave at least two days a week free in which to let your muscles relax.

Once you have had basic tuition, which will enable you to check you are doing things correctly, you can do all of these at home.

Breathlessness on Limited Exertion (Poor Aerobic Performance)

If you get out of breath easily, you should try one of the following:

• Cycling

• Swimming

• Walking

• Jogging

• Dancing

• Skipping

• Any sport that involves rhythmic, continuous activity which places increased demands on the heart and lungs.

If you are a beginner, build up to 20 minutes of continuous activity three times a week.

Aerobic activity can easily be built in to your daily life e.g. by taking a walk every lunch time, or cycling instead of taking a bus or driving.

Lack of Muscular Strength and Poor Muscle Tone

To increase muscle strength and improve muscle tone, try:

• Pilates

• Lotte Berk

• Body sculpting

• Holistix

• Aqua aerobics

• Medau

• Yoga

A minimum of three times a week if possible. If you can only manage once a week at first, that's fine, just build things up gently.

Most of these can be done at home once you have become familiar with the exercises in a class.

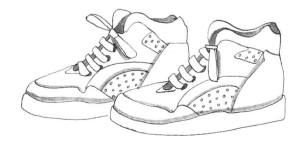

Marked Muscular Tension and Lack of Relaxation

The following forms of exercise help to relax body and mind:

- Yoga

- Pilates

- Medau

- Holistix

- Autogenic training

- Diaphragmatic breathing.

- Any activity you find soothing or relaxing.

Do these exercises any time you feel the need to relax. This could be every day, or depending on your own needs at any time.

There are many audio tapes available which can talk you through a guided relaxation. Other methods of relaxation could be less formal, like going out for a gentle walk, or having a massage.

You will have noticed that some exercise methods appear in different sections under different headings in the tables above. This is because they are methods that have wide-ranging application: they may, for example, improve flexibility *and* induce physical and mental relaxation.

More About Aerobic Exercise

Aerobic activity is any vigorous and rhythmic exercise that conditions the heart and lungs. For it to be most beneficial it needs to be maintained at a level of 60–80 per cent of your heart's maximum capacity for a minimum of twenty minutes at least three times a week. Because aerobic exercise involves the taking in of oxygen to the body, it is very important not to be misled into thinking that you need to push yourself to the point of exhaustion: this is neither healthy nor beneficial.

If exhaustion takes place and you are so breathless that you cannot hold a conversation with ease, this is a sign that you have entered a phase of **anaerobic** activity, which means that your heart and lungs are being deprived of oxygen. Anaerobic exercise has the opposite effect of aerobic activity by slowing down the fat-burning processes of the body, burning more carbohydrates, and eventually diminishing muscle mass. Apart from the stress this sort of activity puts on the body, it is also unlikely that someone who feels wrung out will be motivated to keep on exercising over a long period of time.

Benefits of long-term, sustained aerobic exercise include an increase in overall fitness and energy levels, improved circulation, decreased body fat and improved stamina. Choices of good aerobic exercise include walking at a brisk pace, skipping, cycling, and dancing for sustained periods of time.

Many people are under the false impression that squash is an excellent aerobic exercise: while it may be very enjoyable as a sport, it involves short bursts of activity with a lot of abrupt stopping and starting, rather than sustained aerobic exercise. There is also a high risk of someone entering a phase of anaerobic activity while playing squash without realizing it.

When beginning aerobic exercise, always build up slowly to a sustained activity that you feel comfortable with. Make sure you warm up first, and always slow your pace gradually: never come to an abrupt stop. If you feel dizzy, breathless or nauseated make sure you don't push yourself further, but gently come to a stop.

If you suffer from weak knee and ankle joints or have spinal problems it is best to avoid any aerobic activity that involves putting strain on these areas, such as jogging or skipping. Consider other possibilities such as walking, or swimming (which is excellent because the water supports your joints while they move). When you exercise make sure that the positioning of your shoulders and pelvis feels comfortable to you, and that you do not feel any strain in your lower back.

How Often Should I Exercise?

Ideally you should aim to incorporate some form of exercise into your life each day. This need not be structured exercise in the form of a specific routine, but should be included quite naturally by choosing to take stairs rather than lifts, walking reasonable distances when on errands rather than taking the car, or even getting off the bus one stop before your destination so that you have the chance to walk the extra distance.

It really is just a matter of remembering to do these things in preference to other habits that have become natural over the years. Once you begin to incorporate these small changes into your life, you will find that they quickly become second nature.

The ideas outlined above will give you the framework into which you can add the following, more structured suggestions.

Things To Remember

- Find a good time of day in which to exercise and make it a part of your daily routine. Best of all, find things that you enjoy doing and that become part of your normal daily activities: this way your exercising will be incorporated naturally into your life.

- It doesn't matter what your initial motivation is for taking up more exercise: people do this for all sorts of reasons, such as wanting improve their body shape, to experience higher energy levels, or to find a way of improving their social life. Whatever the reason for beginning, you will quickly realize that the benefits of exercising are as varied as the people who do it.

- If you skip a few days don't feel guilty or demoralized. Part of the excitement and dynamism of life is not knowing what is around the corner, so it is inevitable that we cannot predict what will be happening four weekends ahead at three in the afternoon. If you miss a few days or a week, just pick up where you left off rather than feeling so demoralized that you just can't find the energy to begin again. You will be surprised how quickly you get back into the swing of things.

- Make sure you set yourself goals that are realistic rather than feeling you can achieve everything at once. If you want a better body shape this will take time, but if you have the patience to stick with it you will see the results you want. The same applies to exercising to boost energy levels or to enhance relaxation: pace yourself and assess your progress every three to four weeks rather than every day.

- If you learn to work in harmony with your body's capacity at each stage of fitness, you are far less likely to sustain injury or make yourself feel ill. Work within your own limits, and never feel obliged to overdo things; after all, you are in competition with no one except yourself.

- If you fall into any of the following categories you should get medical advice before beginning any vigorous exercise activity:

  - If you have any history of back trouble or injuries.

  - If you are overweight.

  - If you experience nausea, dizziness or marked breathlessness on exertion.

  - If you are pregnant.

  - If you have not exercised for a long time.

119

Are Special Fitness Clothes Essential?

A lot of people can be put off the idea of exercising because they think it has inevitably to involve large-scale expenditure on designer fitness clothes. For the sort of exercise suggested in the following pages you don't have to dash out and buy the latest fashion in dancewear if you don't want to.

For **stretching exercises** all you will need is something to wear that feels loose and comfortable. Avoid clothes that feel restricting around the waist or under the arms. Trousers or shorts are more practical than skirts, and all-in-one jumpsuits are often excellent for this purpose. If you are considering buying specific items to exercise in, you are likely to find that all-in-one stretch garments are more practical than wearing separate leotards and tights (they are also quicker and easier to get on and off). When buying tights it is a good idea to choose stirrup or footless tights: they help you grip the floor more easily with your feet thus avoiding the possibility of slipping.

Relaxation techniques call for the same requirements as above, with the added consideration that you need to ensure you are warm enough. This is because deep relaxation is accompanied by a significant drop in body temperature, so you need to keep warm and comfortable throughout. Above all, consider that what you wear must be comfortable enough for you to forget about it.

For **aerobic activity** like brisk walking all you will need are comfortable, flat shoes that support your feet well. If you choose to jog you will need trainers designed for that purpose, because well-fitting shoes provide support for the foot and help minimize the risk of injury. Track suits are the most convenient articles of clothing to wear when jogging. A sports bra can also be an asset in making running more comfortable, as well as providing important support for the breasts.

How Essential is it to Warm Up and Cool Down After Exercise?

If you want to get the most out of exercising, you need to know why warming up and a cool down are very important. By limbering up you are far less likely to injure yourself, since many sports injuries happen as a result of exercising muscles that are either too cold and/or insufficiently relaxed. This is especially relevant to stretching exercises, which can be gradually built up in intensity and repetition, as muscles are enabled to take the stretch more easily. Warm-ups are also an excellent way of preparing the mind for exercise as you gently ease into activity: otherwise it can feel like an abrupt shock to the system. On the other hand, if you are just about to go out for a walk there is obviously no need to do any special preparation: just go!

Cooling down is even more essential, especially after any aerobic activity. Always bear in mind that you should never stop vigorous aerobic exercise abruptly, but gradually decrease the pace, regulating your breathing as you do so. As with the warm up, a cool-down period will help in marking the end of your exercise activity, and enable you to feel oriented towards whatever you have to do next. This is especially true after deep relaxation, when you need to resume activity slowly rather than rushing things, otherwise you are likely to lose the be nefits you have gained from being in a state of relaxation.

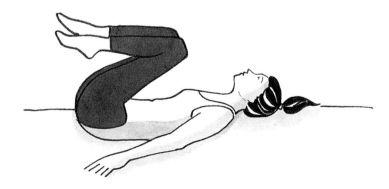

Will Exercise Help Me To Lose Weight?

The rate at which we lose or gain weight is determined by our metabolic rate: in other words, the rate at which we burn up the food we have taken in. If this rate is slow or sluggish, even if the amount of food which is taken in has a low calorific value, any food which is not utilized in energy and heat production will be conserved and laid down as fatty deposits.

If, on the other hand, someone with a high metabolic rate takes in the identical amount of food, they will find their bodies burn up their calorific intake more efficiently, leaving little if any food spare for storage and thus keeping their weight stable. Because of this basic fact, contemporary advice given on weight-reduction increasingly emphasizes the importance of an efficient metabolism, rather than solely concentrating on calorie-controlled diets. It has now become apparent that restricting food intake is not an efficient long-term strategy for effective weight loss. Although diets can initially enable someone to lose weight, most people find they quickly reach a plateau where their weight remains the same, even though they are still severely restricting their intake of food.

In the latter situation, exercising regularly can help speed up metabolic rate, thereby bringing about weight loss and/or improving body shape—*providing* exercise is combined with a diet that is low in fat and sugar but high in complex carbohydrates. For this effect to be maintained it is essential for the exercise to be engaged in regularly: for instance, it is not beneficial to put aside an hour every two weeks, but a minimum of twenty or thirty minutes of aerobic exercise at least three times a week would be excellent.

If exercise becomes a regular feature of life it can have the added bonus of modifying the ratio of muscle to body fat, to the advantage of the former. Although many women find that they look leaner and have a more slender body shape by keeping up regular exercise, they may be surprised to find that their weight has remained the same or even increased by a pound or two. This is because muscle weighs more than fat, so as muscles are toned and firmed they actually start to weigh more than a flabby, out of condition muscle group, while at the same time, paradoxically, inches are melting away from around the waist, hips and thighs.

Is it Better to Attend an Exercise Class or is it Possible to Achieve the Same Effect at Home?

~

At the beginning of selecting an exercise plan, it is worth making time available to attend a class. This ensures that you will have the necessary guidance and advice at the outset which lessens the risk of injury. Once you have become familiar with what is involved, whether or not to attend a class is really down to individual choice.

Some women find they are much more motivated by attending a class, and would find it very hard to maintain the same commitment by relying on self-motivation at home. There can also be a strong element of sociability and conviviality associated with going out to a class which can be missed by someone who works out by themselves. If the exercise programme you choose includes the use of specialized equipment, you will need to find a gym that you feel comfortable with.

Arguments in favour of exercising at home include the freedom of being able to choose when you exercise, the reduction in time spent which can be very attractive to someone who has a busy schedule, and the basic psychological fact that some women do not take well to group activity, but feel much more comfortable with exercising alone.

With the advent of the exercise video, exercising at home has changed. In many ways, video tape has become the bridge between the formality of a class, and the confusion that used to arise from following an exercise book at home. It is essential, however, to point out that some video tapes have recently been severely criticised because they include exercises that may result in injury. If you are concerned about this, it is worth familiarizing yourself with reports that have been published in consumer magazines giving an appraisal of the safety and efficacy of some popular exercise video tapes.

Another way of avoiding this situation is to attend a class for a while. This will give you a chance to evaluate how at ease you feel with the exercise technique you have chosen, and should give you the important guidance and tuition you need to become familiar with how the exercises should be done. This is especially important if you have not exercised for a long time and feel generally unfit. Always choose a small class where the teacher is able to spend time with you, checking that you are doing the exercises correctly. Once you feel at ease and confident with a system of exercise, you can choose whether you want to continue attending a class or get into the habit of exercising at home.

One of the basic advantages of using an informative and safety-conscious video is that, unlike a book, you will be given a good idea of the pace which you should be aiming for, and unlike using an audio cassette, you will also see how the exercise should look when done properly.

What About Exercise Addiction?

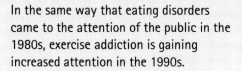

In the same way that eating disorders came to the attention of the public in the 1980s, exercise addiction is gaining increased attention in the 1990s.

In many ways the two phenomena are linked: many women and a growing proportion of men are led to exercise and control their food intake because of a basic dissatisfaction with body image. The common features shared by both groups include:

• Low self-esteem.

• Tendencies to perfectionism and competitiveness.

• Fear of failure.

• Desire to establish control.

• Difficulties in establishing and maintaining close relationships.

Exercise addiction can be seen as the legacy of the extremely tough and competitive atmosphere of exercise in the 1980s. Addiction to exercise involves such a degree of disruption in someone's life that it can only be supported by isolation from friends and family. Just as an anorexic or bulimic will go to any lengths to maintain their 'habit', the obsessive runner or jogger will put exercising before any other priority. Even injuries will not prevent the true addict: there are numerous anecdotes of runners who feel compelled to run even when in severe pain.

Exercise addiction is an excellent example of how something that is health-promoting can become the opposite if perception of it gets out of balance. Once it has reached the obsessional stage, addiction to exercise has become destructive rather than life affirming.

With the gentler and more rounded approach to exercise in the 1990s, it is to be hoped that exercise addiction will seem very out of step with the basic philosophy of holism, with its emphasis on supporting the body rather than subduing it. Sadly, addiction to exercise does the very opposite to a balanced and integrated approach: it creates stress rather than diminishing it, especially if exercise is denied for any length of time.

Exercise in itself is not the problem: it is the attitude that is brought to it that determines whether things are in balance or not. The following features are often indicators that someone is experiencing difficulties with regard to exercise, and that it is entering a phase of imbalance:

• Giving total priority to exercise at the expense of social and family life.

• Feeling profound guilt, anger, or extreme physical unease if some-thing happens to prevent exercising.

• Constantly pushing the boundaries and exercise goals further and further, especially if this is linked with restricting food intake.

• Increasing dissatisfaction with body image.

• Increased isolation and self-preoccupation.

Exercise is a tool that we can use in the same way as good nutrition or relaxation techniques to enhance our lives and make them more rounded, but an obsessional approach *prevents* us from experiencing good emotional and physical health. The answer lies not in avoiding exercise, but in establishing a new perspective and model for exercising that celebrates its positive and life-enhancing qualities.

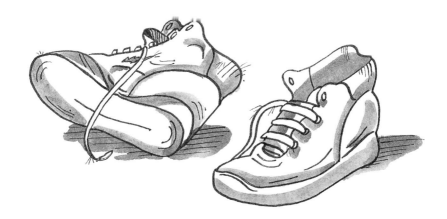

Exercise Systems to Choose From

In this section you will find a quick tour of some of the exercise systems available to you. A variety of well-known techniques have been included, but this is in no way intended to be an exhaustive list. This section will give you a basic idea of what is involved in each system, but does not imply a personal endorsement of any one method.

Exercises That Aid Flexibility and Improve Muscle Tone

The Pilates Method

Although the Pilates method was developed as far back as the 1920s, it is a form of exercise that has increasingly broad application and popularity today. Originally designed as a physiotherapeutic tool, Pilates concentrates on encouraging the development of a fine sense of body awareness while exercising.

By tailoring basic exercise techniques to individual needs, Pilates teaching does not force anyone to repeat a posture that they feel unhappy or uncomfortable with. The result is an exercise technique that builds muscular strength, reduces stress, increases flexibility, and encourages awareness of harmful postural habits that have been built up over the years.

In many ways, Pilates is the opposite of the high-impact, competitive, communal classes of the 1980s. Because successful use of the technique involves precise working of specific muscles for a limited number of repetitions, tuition will be given on an individual basis within the context of a small class. Although weak muscles are being strengthened and tight muscles are stretched, Pilates will not lead to the development of a bulky outline. In fact, the overall effect as muscle tone is improved should be that the body appears taller and more slender as it settles into improved alignment.

Because the exercises demand a high level of concentration, they help someone escape the trap of mindlessly executing high repetitions of exercises in the hope that they may be doing some good. In Pilates the degree of attention that is brought to the exercises encourages someone to focus on how their body is reacting, and brings about a keener sense of the benefits they are gaining from exercising.

The following information is based on an article entitled 'Take Control' (*Here's Health*, June 1992, pp. 35–37).

Warm Up

Stand with feet about a hip width apart with knees relaxed. Rest your fingers on your upper abdomen. When you breathe out feel the stomach pulling up as your shoulders and tail bone drop. Do this four times, each time being conscious of the alignment of your pelvis.

Arm Circles

Circle one arm forward four times while breathing in through the mouth and out through the nose. Repeat the same breathing pattern while you circle the same arm in the reverse direction (backwards) for another count of four. Do the same with the other arm.

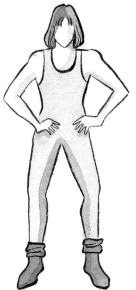

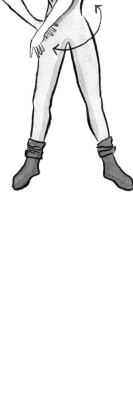

Shoulder Lifts

Lift both shoulders, squeeze, hold for a few seconds and gently relax them down. Do this four times. Lift the left shoulder for a total of four counts, and repeat with the right shoulder. Slowly and gently turn your head from side to side without straining, pushing or moving your shoulder.

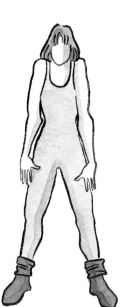

Stomach Tighteners

1. Lie on the floor with your knees bent and feet about a hip width apart flat on the floor. Support your head by cradling it in your hands while you press your lower back into the floor. From this position, curve your body forward, lifting one leg in a slow and controlled way as you breathe in. Pause with your leg in a lifted position, then let it descend gently, breathing out and pulling the stomach up. Repeat for a total of five counts on each side.

2. Still supporting your neck and shoulders with your hands, relax your lower back into the floor, bringing your knees in towards your chest as you flatten your stomach pulling it in against your spine, and feel your middle back supported by the floor.

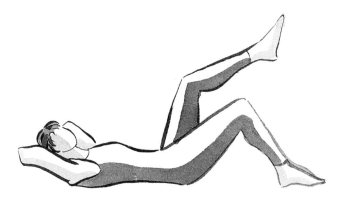

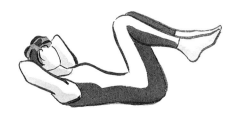

As you maintain this position, extend one leg until it is straight as you breathe out, keeping the other leg bent. Repeat with alternating legs for 10 counts, making sure you hold the stomach in as you repeat each movement. Do this exercise slowly and stop if you experience any sense of strain in your back.

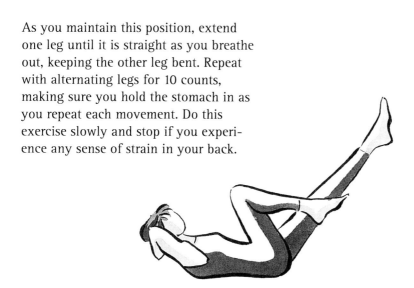

For the following arm exercises you will need to use hand-held weights of approximately 1–2 pounds ($^1/_2$–1 kg). You can buy weights at a shop which specializes in fitness clothes and accessories or you can use a medium-sized can of food which weighs approximately the same amount.

Arm Exercises Using Weights

Shoulders
Lie on your back with knees bent and feet a hip width apart flat on the floor. Support your head with folded towel or a flat cushion. Holding the weights, extend your arms at shoulder level straight above your chest without locking your elbows. As you breathe in open your arms slowly, extending them gently to the sides as far as they will comfortably go. As you breathe out, gently and slowly raise your arms to the position in which you started. Repeat 10 times Relax your back into the floor as you do this exercise.

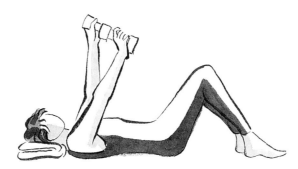

Inner Thighs

Lie on one side supporting your head on your hand. Keeping your underneath leg stretched, bend your top leg in front of you, letting it rest on a cushion or folded towel. When you breathe out lift the straight leg as far as your stomach muscles will allow. Hold for a couple of seconds, then slowly lower the leg. Repeat on each side ten times.

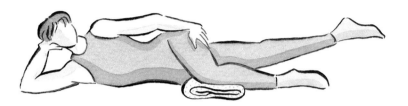

Buttocks

Lie on your stomach, resting your head on folded arms, with a folded towel under your stomach. Pull your stomach into your spine as you tighten your buttock muscles. Bend one knee, lift it an inch holding for a few seconds, straighten the leg, and gently ease it down again. Do this ten times on each side. Take care that you do not arch your back: your stomach should hold the position without straining your back.

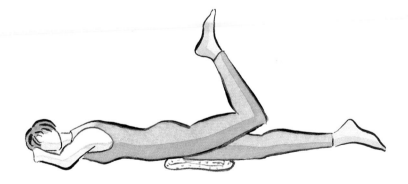

Medau

It is no surprise that the Medau technique can also be referred to as **The Art of Energy**, since it is a comprehensive method of exercising that aims to boost energy levels, using exercises that promote strength and stamina, flexibility, and harmony between body and mind through relaxation.

Medau dates from the turn of the century and was developed by Hinrich Medau as a system of movement designed to liberate the body from repetitive and rigid exercises. In freeing the body from a mechanical approach to exercise, Medau drew inspiration for his system from the fluid movements of athletes, animals and dancers such as Isadora Duncan. What ensued was a system of exercise that encouraged a range of graceful, flowing movements which increased body awareness, helped develop and maintain good posture, relaxed body and mind, and encouraged an intuitive pleasure in responding to rhythm.

Although developed so long ago (Medau founded his own training college in 1929), Medau fits in well with the current need to discover an approach to exercise which is rounded and geared to individual needs. Age is no barrier to practising Medau: children can benefit from the method as much as women and men in their sixties. You can concentrate on the aspect of Medau to which you want to give priority, but teachers suggest that if you do the full range of Medau exercises you should enjoy a rounded experience of exercise which benefits body and

mind. For further information, see *Medau: The Art of Energy* by Lucy Jackson (Thorsons).

Warm Up

1. Stand with your feet about a hip width apart. With your toes keeping contact with the floor, lift each heel alternately as you remain on the spot. As you gain momentum and raise each foot off the floor, lift each elbow forwards and back alternately in a swinging movement in time with your feet.

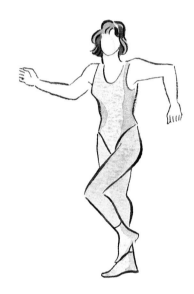

2. Step to one side and bring the other foot across to meet it, bending your knees slightly as your foot moves to the side. Continue by moving in the opposite direction in the same way. Repeat this movement eight times on each side.

3. Go back to stepping on the spot, using your arms and legs in a more vigorous way than when you began. Then with your arms at hip-level tug your clenched fists towards your hips, turning a little with your weight on the opposite leg. Do this for a total of sixteen counts (eight on each side).

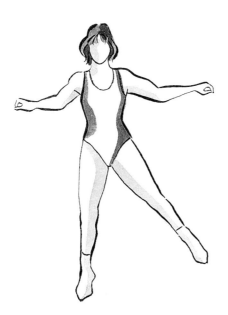

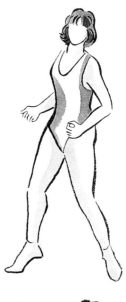

4. Keeping your hands clenched, make small punches away from your body at shoulder-level for the same number of counts at either side. Return to stepping, gradually bringing the pace down until you return to lifting the heels off the floor slowly and gently. Breathe regularly, deeply and rhythmically, gradually coming to a halt when your breathing has returned to normal.

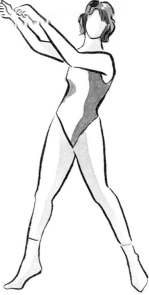

Stretching
Preparation

Check your posture by standing with your feet a hip-distance apart. As you are standing, experience the length and extension of your body from your neck to the base of your spine. Move your head gently from side to side then tilt gently and slowly, backwards and forwards. Check that your posture is in alignment by lightly placing your hands on your head, shoulders and hips in turn.

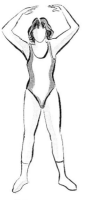
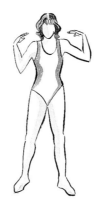
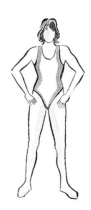

Back and Upper Arms

1. Raise your arms, bend your elbows and press the shoulder blades together, flattening your upper back as you do so. Do this four times. Drop your hands behind you and press the shoulder blades together once again.

2. Press your hands on your knees, tightening your abdominal muscles as you curve your middle back. Hold this position for as long as feels comfortable without straining. Lift your upper body out from the hips in order to relieve pressure in your lower back.

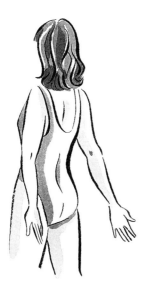
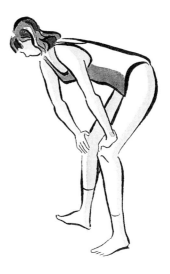

133

3. Keeping your knees bent, lift your body with arms raised keeping your elbows bent. Press round into a side twist, lifting upwards from the hips allowing the leg on the opposite side of the twist to lift and follow the movement around. Repeat on the other side.

4. Stand with your feet apart, checking that your toes and knees are pointing in the same direction. Press down into a half-squatting position with your hands resting on your upper thighs just below your hips. Feel as though you are about to sit. Then pull up strongly through your whole back as you tighten your pelvic floor muscles, making sure you also pull in your stomach muscles. If you find it difficult to tighten your pelvic floor muscles with your feet apart, try pulling up with your feet closer together.

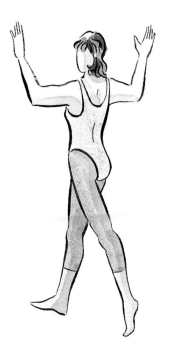

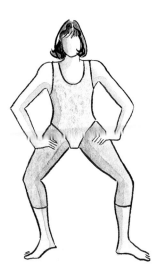

Strengthening Abdominal Muscles

1. Gently lower yourself to the floor until you are sitting with a straight back and both legs extended in front of you. Bend one leg towards your body and put a hand under one knee and the other over it. Keeping this position with your buttocks tight and your abdominals held in, lean back slowly. Change legs and pull up strongly with the other leg. Crossing your feet, squeeze your thighs and muscles of the pelvic floor, pushing both your heels down.

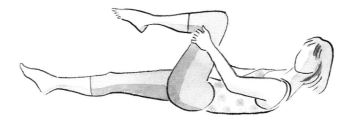

2. Stretch out and turn over to face downwards with your legs stretched long behind you. Keeping your legs extended lift your feet roughly two inches off the floor and 'walk' slowly using small steps. Avoid straining your back by not lifting your heels too high, and keep your head down to avoid straining your neck.

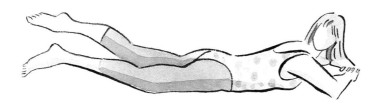

3. In the same position, try lifting your feet with your knees apart. As with the previous exercise, do not lift your legs too high. This is very strenuous, and you will need to roll over on to your back and rest with your knees bent to relax afterwards.

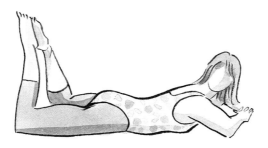

The Lotte Berk Technique

Based on a combination of modern ballet, yoga and orthopaedic exercise, the Lotte Berk technique concentrates on firming the body and producing a shapely outline. The technique works from the premise that daily exercise is necessary in order to achieve and maintain a supple, strong, and firm body at any age. Multiple repetitions are not called for: it is more important to do a small number of exercises correctly on a regular basis.

The core of the technique rests on the concept of 'rolling in'. This is achieved by lying on the floor with knees bent, rolling the small of the back into the floor. This ensures that the back is absolutely flat and maintains contact with the floor while exercising. If you are doing this correctly, there should be no gap between the hollow of your back and the floor. By keeping 'rolled in' while doing the stomach exercises you should ensure that you do not suffer back ache or hurt your spine. As with most of the exercises mentioned in this section, maintaining correct posture is essential in order to get the maximum benefits from exercising.

If your muscles ache after exercising this is a sign that areas which have been underused are beginning to wake up: don't give in to the temptation to give up at this stage, but continue to exercise regularly and you should find that you ache less as your muscles gain in strength and flexibility.

Always make sure that you spend time warming up before you begin any other exercises: this is essential in order to avoid straining or tearing cold or under-used muscles. Warming up boosts the circulation and loosens up the body, preparing it for more specific exercises. For further information, see *The Lotte Berk Method of Exercise* by Lotte Berk and Jean Prince (Quartet).

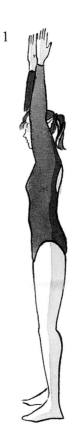

1

Warm Up

Stand with your feet hip distance apart with your hands at your sides. Keeping your elbows straight, stretch your arms above your head. Bending your knees, bring your arms forward and downwards in a sweeping motion, as you bend your body forwards, until they are swept behind your body. Swing your arms forward as you come up again, sweeping your arms behind your head and bending your elbows. Make this a fluid, continuous movement, repeating it ten times.

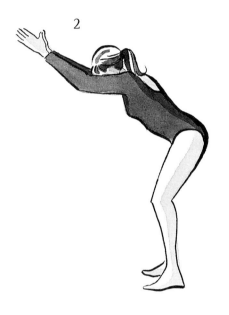

2

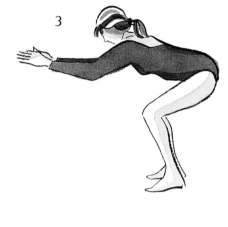

3

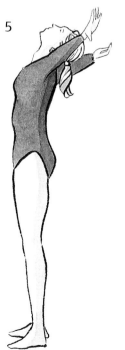

5

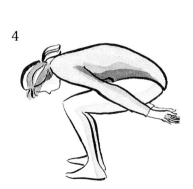

4

Thigh Lifts

Holding on to a firm surface with your right hand (this could be a heavy chair, radiator, or even a kitchen sink!) stand sideways on, extending and raising your left leg to the side as you steady yourself with your left arm extended straight out at shoulder level. Bending over your left leg slightly, bend and stretch your extended leg ten times, making sure you stretch as hard and fully as you can. Relax the leg and repeat on the other side.

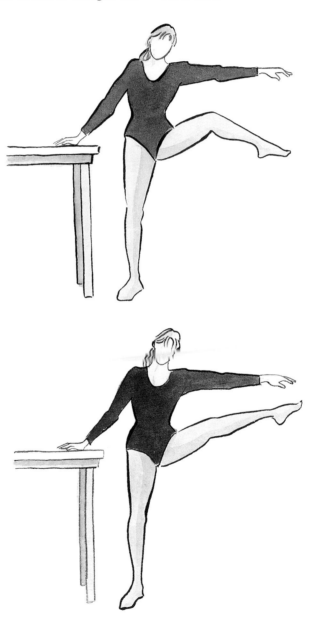

Stomach Tighteners

1. Lie down with your knees bent and your feet a hip width apart. Stretch your arms behind your head, and roll your back into the floor so that your lower back maintains contact with the carpet. Lift your head and shoulders off the floor as you grip your thighs, keeping your elbows out to the sides.

Let go of your thighs as you keep your head and shoulders raised, hold this position for a second before relaxing. Repeat five times. If you are doing this exercise correctly, you should feel the muscles working around the base of your rib-cage.

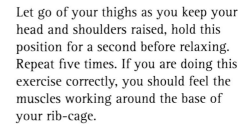

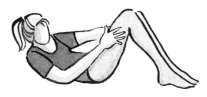

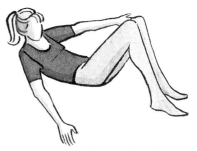

2. Start by lying down with knees bent and feet resting on the floor. Roll your back into the floor and lift your head and shoulders off the floor, tilting your chin towards your chest rather like a baby in the womb. Keeping this position, with your back 'rolled in', rest your hands on your knees. Lift your feet a few inches off the floor and slowly rock backwards and forwards. As you roll forwards, briefly take your hands off your knees and

extend your arms forwards. This should be a very small, controlled movement: your upper back should only move a few inches from the floor as you come up. Hold on once again to your knees with your hands as you roll back. As you do this exercise avoid tightening your buttock muscles. Repeat this five times, gradually building up the number of repetitions as you get stronger.

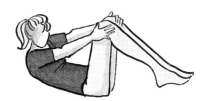

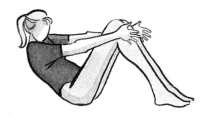

Cool Down Stretch

Sit down with your legs apart and stretched out on each side. Stretch your arms straight up towards the ceiling and flex your feet so that they come up a little off the floor. Turn towards your right foot and stretch out; taking hold of your right foot, move your head down towards your knee making sure you do not strain. Come back to centre, sit tall and repeat on the other side.

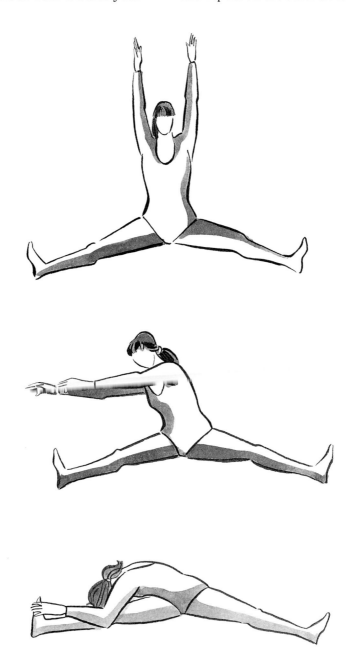

Holistix

The Holistix approach to exercise emphasizes the role of bodily movement in helping us achieve a balance between body and mind. By conditioning and looking after our bodies it is possible to discover a new sense of confidence as body shape changes and strength and flexibility increase.

Holistix is more than an exercise regime, since it encourages someone to review the quality of their life as a whole with respect to diet, health problems and emotional well-being. Exercise fits appropriately within this context as an aid to relaxation, increased vitality, and well-being.

Exercises are taught in conjunction with clear advice about how to breathe to get the maximum value from each exercise. Postural correction is also emphasized to lessen the risk of injury. In class the exercises are tailored to each individual's needs so that as much benefit as possible can be derived from the movements. This also prevents the risk of exercise becoming routine and fixed, since there is scope for changes within the basic format of the exercise postures. For further information see *Holistix* by Carole Caplin (Sidgwick & Jackson)

Warm Up

Standing with your feet wide apart and pointing straight ahead, put your hands on your shoulders as you bring your pelvis forward and pull your stomach into your back. Keeping your chin up, pull your elbows back as you breathe in. With your elbows pointing up to the ceiling and keeping your buttock muscles tight, release the elbows forward and down as you breathe out through your mouth. Repeat this movement eight times.

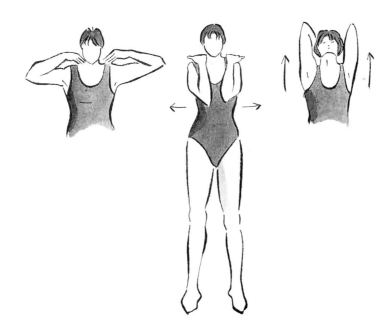

Toning Exercises for Calves, Thighs and Buttocks

1. Using a surface at waist level to hold on to (the back of a chair, radiator, or banister will be suitable provided they give you a firm, immovable surface to support yourself), stand with your feet together and legs straight. Standing facing your barre, pull upwards from your waist, elongating your spine and neck without straining. Keeping this position, lift your heels off the ground as you keep your feet together. Hold for a second, then let your heels down without touching the ground. Do this twice in the position described, twice with feet turned out and heels touching, twice with feet parallel and apart, and twice with feet turned out and apart.

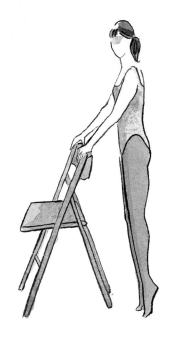

2. Calf Stretch: Shake out and relax your legs. Starting from the same position with your body pulled up and hands resting on a support, bring your right foot forwards keeping your left foot back. Keeping your body upright, and your feet facing forward, bend your front knee and push forward from your pelvis, without collapsing your body into the stretch. Keep your back leg straight with your heel keeping contact with the floor. Make sure you keep your left hip pushed forward so that your pelvis keeps straight. Do this for a count of eight. Repeat the same posture on the other side, keeping your body pulled up.

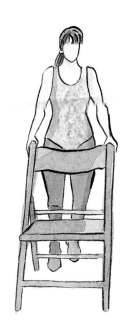

Exercises to Encourage Mobility of Hip Joints

1. Kneel down until you are on all fours with your arms straight and at right-angles to your body with palms of your hands flat on the floor. Have your hands sufficient distance away from your hips to allow your shoulders to relax away from your ears.

Keeping this position, lift your right knee, keeping your leg bent as you point your right foot. Ensure that you keep your knee higher than your foot as you bring your right knee forward and back eight times. Relax in between, then repeat the same exercise on the left side.

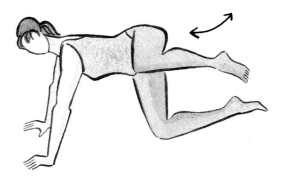

2. Starting from the same position, bring your right knee up, still checking that your knee is higher than your foot on that side, and lift the knee up and down eight times. Relaxing in between, repeat on the left side.

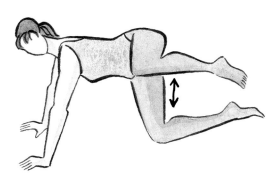

Stomach Exercises

1. Begin by lying on your back, knees bent, feet wide apart, and feet flat on the floor. Supporting your head with your hands, squeeze your pelvic muscles tight, keeping the small of your back pressed into the floor as you raise your head and shoulders a small distance off the floor. Breathing regularly and deeply, hold this position for a count of four before you gently release your head and shoulders back to the floor. Do this four times. Relax by cradling your bent knees against your chest, pulling them towards your chest.

2. Sit with a straight back, knees bent, feet flat on the floor, and arms extended straight ahead at shoulder-level. Slowly lower yourself back on to the floor keeping your arms straight and extended as you do so. Then bring yourself slowly up, keeping your back rounded and chin tucked in to the chest. As you sit up make sure that you open your rib cage and chest, keeping your shoulders back and down. Repeat twenty times, making sure you avoid:

- Arching your back as you come up or go down.

- Landing with force.

- Using your arms to bring you up.

- Straining your neck.

- Hunching your shoulders up to your ears.

Relax by cradling your knees once again.

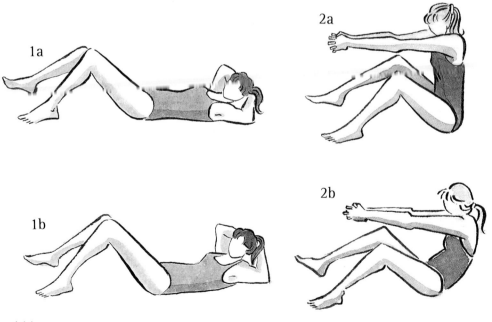

Exercises That Encourage Flexibility and Relaxation

Yoga

Hatha Yoga is the form of Yoga with which most of us in the West are familiar. While it requires stamina and mental concentration to hold a Yoga posture for any length of time, it is also acknowledged as an excellent way of enabling the mind to relax and unwind: when practised regularly, Yoga leads not only to physical flexibility and strength but also to an understanding of how breathing techniques contribute to relaxation. Yoga is quite challenging, therefore, but the rewards can be startling in terms of increased energy or well-being.

Yoga is an especially attractive option to those of us who have been put off exercising in youth by the competitive aspects of sport, and its often spartan conditions. In Yoga, you are in competition with no one, and never need to force yourself beyond a point that you feel comfortable with. It is also worth bearing in mind that most exercises can be modified for those who may have limitations in flexibility or fitness.

Furthermore, because Yoga has at its centre the philosophy of harmony and balance between mind and body, the resulting sense of body awareness often guards against someone injuring themselves by pushing their bodies too far.

Because the postures are executed slowly, there is less chance of injury from jerking or pulling muscles violently. Establishing a good breathing technique also helps guard against injury as you learn to breathe in to a posture, rather than forcing into a movement with tense muscles.

Most important of all, Yoga relaxation and breathing will help you relax and unwind if you are feeling stressed. Once you master how to use your breathing as an aid to relaxation, you can use it at any time you feel anxious or overstretched. For further information, see *Wake Up to Yoga* and *Keep Up with Yoga* by Lyn Marshall (Ward Lock).

The Refresher

(See illustrations on p. 146.) Stand with your feet about two feet apart and your hands at your sides and breathe in through your nose. Gently and slowly allow your body to relax forward, letting your arms and hands hang loosely as you breathe out. Soften, or even bend the knees, and let gravity take you forward until you are hanging loosely from your hips with your fingers brushing the floor: do not strain, but only come down as far as feels comfortable to you. Hold this position for a count of ten, and then slowly come up, gradually lifting your head last. (NB Do not take your head lower than your hips if you have a heart or blood pressure condition.)

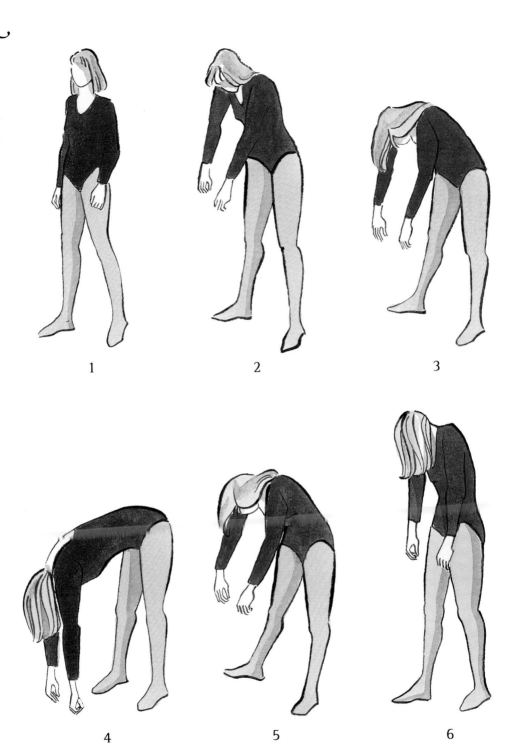

1

2

3

4

5

6

The Triangle

Begin from the same position with feet a leg-length apart. Bring your arms up to shoulder-level keeping them straight. Maintaining straight elbows, slowly lengthen the spine and bend over to the left side. Allow your left hand to touch the left leg wherever it can comfortably reach. Lift the right hand to the ceiling with arm straight and palm facing downward. Hold this position for a count of five without straining, then gradually return to centre. Pause, and then repeat on the other side. Repeat once more on both sides, taking care to breathe evenly as you move in and out of the posture. Take in a deep breath as you raise your arms and breathe out as you go over to one side. Breathe smoothly as you hold the posture. (NB Take care to bend to the side and avoid twisting the hips. Be especially careful to avoid strain if you have back trouble, and practise close to a wall if your balance is weak.)

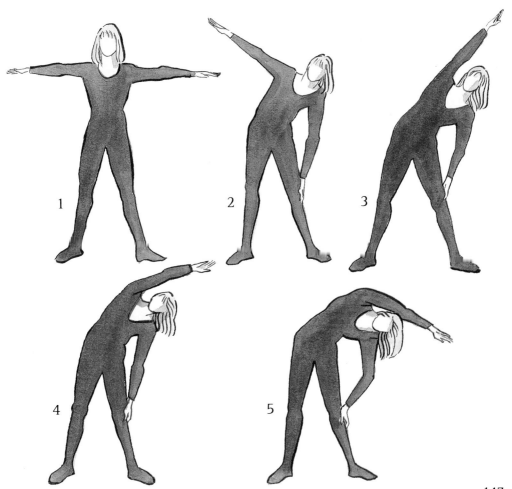

The Cat

Come down on all fours with your hands beneath your shoulders, knees under your hips. Slowly arch your back, breathing out as you move, tucking your tail under, with your head hanging loosely out of your neck. Now breathe in, and return slowly to a level position before you move your buttocks toward the ceiling, creating a hollow in your mid-back. Raise your head and hold for a count of five, breathing smoothly, before repeating the whole sequence again. Repeat up to six times. (NB Take care with this posture if you have a history of back problems, and avoid it altogether if you suffer from rheumatoid arthritis.)

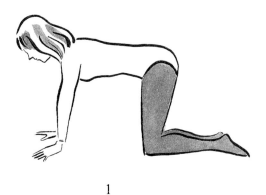

1

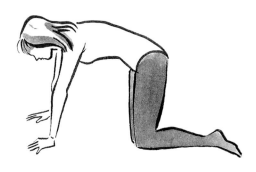

2

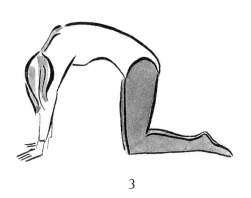

3

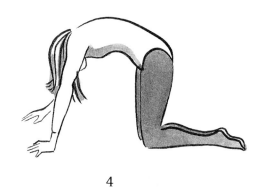

4

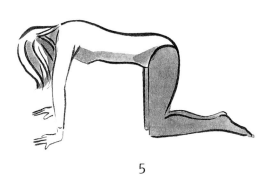

5

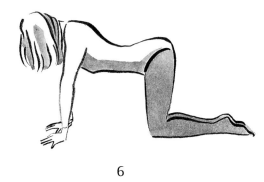

6

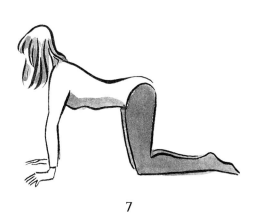

7

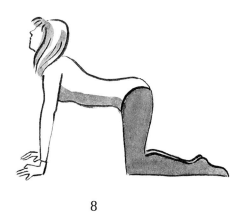

8

149

The Cobra

Lie on your stomach feeling fully relaxed with your arms at your sides. Let your heels fall open and consciously relax your fingers and hands. Rest your forehead gently on the floor as you bring your feet together. Place your hands underneath your shoulders with the palms of your hands and your elbows resting on the floor. Raise your face slowly towards the ceiling until your back is comfortably arched. Do not strain in this position but feel you can maintain the posture without shaking or breathing irregularly. Hold for a count of five, and come down slowly by bending your elbows as you keep your head back. Gently bring your forehead down until it is resting on the floor again, and bring your hands back to your sides. Rest, and repeat the whole movement once again. Remember to keep your elbows on the floor if you have back trouble, and keep your head level. Try to use your back muscles to lift into the posture, using hands only for support.

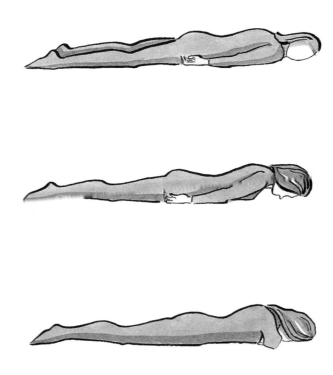

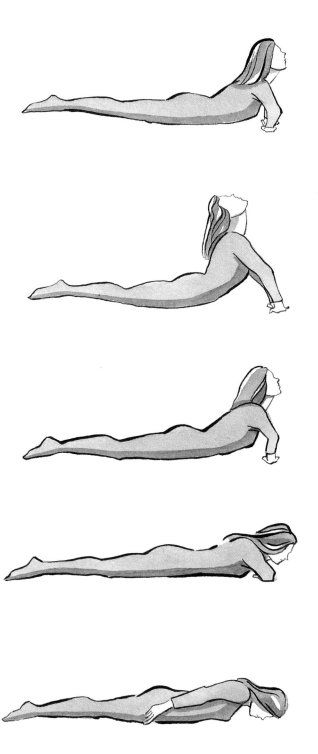

Thigh Stretch

Sit on the floor with your knees bent and the soles of your feet together. Holding your ankles in your hands and keeping your back as straight as possible gently push your knees down, hold for a couple of seconds, then let your knees come up again. Repeat this movement five times.

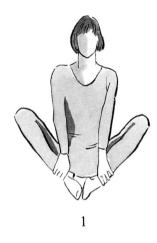

1

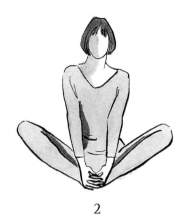

2

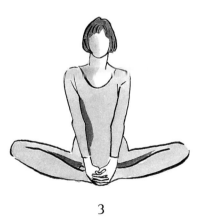

3

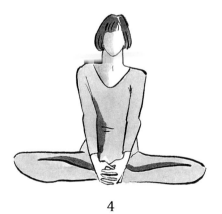

4

The Corpse

Lie down with your arms at your side and your legs a little apart. Relax your leg muscles, letting your feet fall gently apart. Move your arms away from your body and rest your hands on their backs. Allow your fingers to curl inwards as your arms relax. Gently lengthen your neck, tilting your chin forward. Now check the head moves easily from side to side (you may need to rest your head on a small cushion). Close your eyes and relax the muscles of your face. Your mouth may drop open slightly as you let go of the tension in your jaw. Gently slow down your breathing without forcing it, letting each breath flow without strain. Focus on the rise and fall of your navel, relaxing any areas where you feel tension or discomfort. Stay in this position for as long as you feel comfortable. When you are ready, do not get up quickly, but slowly bring your attention back to your surroundings, gently stretching each part of your body and opening your eyes. Sit up slowly to ensure that you do not feel dizzy or disoriented.

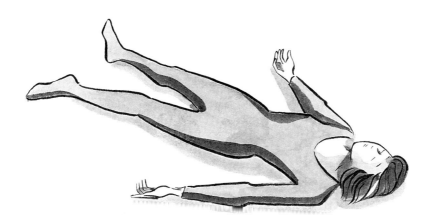

Techniques That Encourage Postural Awareness

The Alexander Technique

Although not strictly speaking an exercise system, the Alexander Technique is relevant to any discussion about body awareness through movement. The technique can be used by anyone to enable them to feel more at ease with their body and to help them take notice of the postural habits they have built up over the years.

Through the technique many people discover an awareness of the way their posture reflects how they feel, especially when under stress. By breaking these habits and opening up the possibility of change, the Alexander Technique can enable someone to break habitual behaviour patterns. By watching our physical reactions to other people and to events we perceive as threatening or difficult, we can learn a lot about how we cope in these situations and decide for ourselves if another way might not be better for us.

These insights can also be of immense value in making us more aware of how our bodies respond to exercise movements, thus enriching our experience while we exercise, and making injury through forcing our bodies into inappropriate postures less likely.

How Emotions Affect Our Posture

Next time you're feeling anxious or stressed, watch what is happening to your body. You will probably find that the muscles in your neck and upper back are tight, your hands may be clenched, and your jaw is likely to be locked shut. If you feel depressed, your shoulders will droop and everything is likely to feel as if it is sagging to the ground. Since maintaining these postural distortions uses up a great deal of energy, the chances are that you will also be feeling weary and lethargic.

That is the negative side of the picture; however, if we reverse it, we can discover how consciousness of our postural habits can help us in situations which are anxious or depressing. By loosening up, relaxing, and becoming more in tune with postural responses, we often find that we can combat feelings of anxiety

or depression. In other words, if we can influence our posture by how we feel, we can equally affect how we feel by altering our posture.

Long-established postural habits take a long time to break. The important thing is to become aware that we can use our bodies to help us through situations of crisis by becoming aware of the signals they are sending us, rather than constantly bracing ourselves, and then wondering later why we feel so exhausted and tense.

Learning to Relax

Benefits of Relaxation

As the pace of life speeds up we need to make space for our minds and bodies to unwind. If we do this, the benefits are enormous: we can think more clearly and creatively, energy levels are higher, and we will generally experience a marked sense of well-being and vitality.

In the same way that our bodies need to rest in order to recharge themselves for the demands they face on a day to day basis, our minds also need time to offload the pressures and strains involved in a hectic day.

Ways of Setting About It

Make sure you get the amount of sleep you need: this will vary for each individual, but most people are aware of the amount of refreshing sleep they require in order to function at their optimum level. If you are having problems sleeping, consider the following:

- Cut down caffeine intake: strong coffee and tea are stimulants that cause wakefulness, palpitations, and sensations of being jittery and on-edge. Avoid caffeine completely in the evenings, and drink soothing warm beverages instead, such as Chamomile tea. Remember that many soft fizzy drinks such as cola contain caffeine too.

- Avoid working late: working until it's time to go to bed is one of the biggest contributors to insomnia. If your mind is still actively working on a problem it becomes almost impossible to switch off.

- Do something you know you find relaxing for an hour or two before bed. This could be anything from watching a favourite video to having a warm bath, or anything else you find relaxing for you.

- Make sure your curtains block out light adequately.

- Regular exercise that involves activities in the open air will do a great deal to help you relax when you need to.

- Correct breathing is an important aid to relaxation: learning to breathe from the diaphragm will help considerably (see section on breathing, page 112).

- Combine things that contribute to your feeling relaxed: for example, you can practise relaxing breathing in the bath or while you listen to soothing music.

- Use aromatherapy creatively: oils can be used in massage, in the bath, or burnt in special holders to scent your room. Oils to consider: Neroli, Narcissus, Rose, or Geranium.

- Learn to be aware of your body and the signals it will send you when things are getting stressed. Tell-tale signs include:

  - Any feelings of tension or stiffness in your neck.

  - Tightness in the jaw (especially if you find yourself holding your breath and clenching your teeth when you are trying to get to sleep).

  - Palpitations (consciousness of your heart beating fast).

  - Muscular stiffness and tension anywhere.

  - Heartburn, indigestion or lack of appetite.

  - Irritability or tearfulness without explanation.

Relaxation Techniques

You may not need to use a specific technique in order to unwind: some of the suggestions given above may be enough on their own. However, here are some of the best approaches if you need help in learning to relax.

Autogenic Training

Autogenic training enables someone to exercise control over feelings of anxiety or panic, and is conducive to states of deep relaxation. By mastering the technique, involuntary functions of the body can be affected. Good examples of these would include control over pulse rate, heartbeat, or breathing rate.

In order to learn how to practise the technique it is important to be trained by a skilled practitioner rather than attempting autogenic training by yourself. The reason for this is simple: learning the technique involves mastering six simple mental exercises involving suggestion that certain sensations are being experienced, such as a sensation of warmth, heaviness, or calmness. Reactions may surface in response to autogenics that need the support and skill of a practitioner at various stages.

Once mastered, autogenic training can be used to affirm positively your natural abilities when you are in a deeply relaxed state. You can practice the technique anywhere you feel comfortable and relaxed, and it does not involve any difficult postures or instructions. However, you will need to practice regularly and develop skills of physical observation as you experience different sensations in your relaxed state.

Simple Steps to Relaxation

If you feel you would like to try some very simple exercises in addition to the basic advice outlined above, the following will be helpful. Make sure you have at least thirty minutes when you know you will be free of interruption.

- Dress in loose comfortable clothes that do not make you feel restricted.

- The room needs to be warm but not stuffy. Remember that your body temperature will drop when you relax and that you want to avoid feeling uncomfortably chilled.

- Lie on your back with knees bent, feet about a foot apart. With one hand on your belly feel the breath moving from your upper chest into your abdomen on the in-breath, and leaving in reverse order on the out-breath.

- The breathing shouldn't feel forced: let it take its own rhythm and establish its own regularity. All you need to do is observe it. (For more advice on breathing from the diaphragm see the earlier section on First Steps in Breathing Technique, page 112.)

- Once you feel you are breathing from the area around your navel, gently relax your legs to the floor, letting your feet fall apart gently. You can also relax your arms, letting your hand rest lightly with their backs on the floor.

- Begin by bringing your attention to your head and face. Beginning with your scalp, imagine relaxing this area by consciously letting go of any tension you feel there. Move down to your forehead, again observing any tightness that you feel there, and consciously letting go.

- Move down your face this way, concentrating on any area that is holding a lot of tension. Feel the relaxation enter your eyes, nose, cheeks, jaw, lips and throat. Your mouth may hang open slightly as you relax which is fine.

- Carry on this process for each area of your body in turn: from the neck, to the shoulders, the arms, the chest, abdomen, buttocks, thighs, knees, calves, ankles and feet. Always spend more time on any area that feels tight and resistant to relaxation.

- You should now feel fully relaxed and comfortable. Bring your attention once more to your breathing without affecting what is happening to it, and you will find that it has slowed down of its own accord.

- As you observe the breath, visualize energy or light entering your body on the in-breath, and tiredness leaving your body on the out-breath. You can modify these images to anything that you feel is appropriate for you and with which you feel at ease.

- Continue to breathe in this way, feeling the relaxation deepen for as long as you feel you want to continue.

- When you are ready, gradually think about bringing your attention back to your surroundings. Move your hands and feet gently, stretching and flexing them. If you feel you want to, start to stretch your whole body, comparing how you feel now with the way you felt before this relaxation exercise.

- Last of all, open your eyes slowly. Avoid sitting up too quickly, but roll gently on to your side when you are ready, and then move to a sitting position.

This is just one basic exercise in relaxation. There are countless variations available, which you can buy on audio tape or video. Experiment with a number of different approaches until you find one that works for you. In the same way that you must find the type of exercise activity that suits you as an individual, the same is true of relaxation.

Always remember that, in order to relax, you don't have to have endless time available. Just as exercise can be incorporated into your daily routine, make time to do things that are relaxing for you. Use your imagination and follow your instincts; after all, advice can only take you so far, and only you can know what feels good to you.

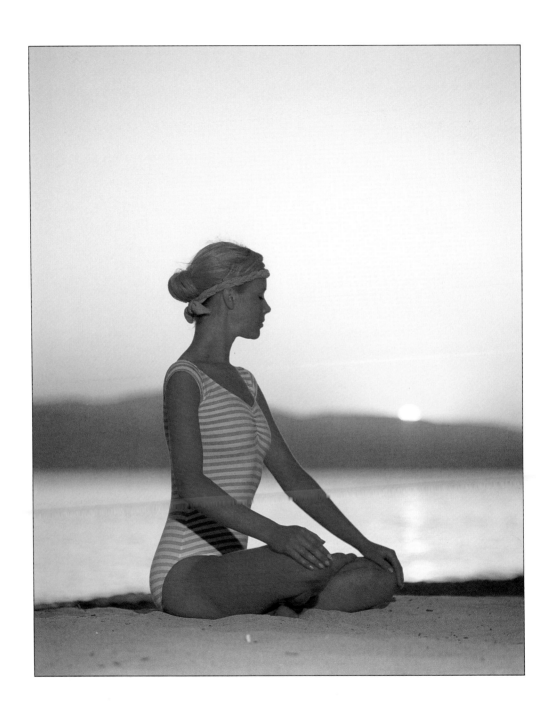

CHAPTER SEVEN

The Mind/Body Link:

Feeling Good, Looking Good

The Importance of Well-Being and Self-Esteem

In order to maximize our potential for vitality and vibrancy we need to look beyond surface appearance and consider underlying emotions such as anxiety, lack of confidence or depression. However much attention we pay to skin care, make-up or designer clothes, these will only provide a superficial veneer of style or sophistication: on their own they cannot give us confidence or a sense of self-worth.

These feelings are experienced when we relax and try as far as possible to accept ourselves with all our positive and negative qualities: in other words, when we enjoy harmony and balance on mental, physical and emotional levels. Once we see ourselves realistically and without exaggerating our faults, we can begin to evaluate our potential and set achievable goals. For goals to be mean-ingful, they have to be realistic: there is little point in starving ourselves to get into a size eight dress if we are naturally

comfortable and feel at our best in a steady size twelve. Unreachable goals will only result in frustration and disappointment: attainable and successfully maintainable ones will boost self-esteem and overall confidence.

These goals will vary according to our individual personality and can range from learning to drive, exploring a fresh exercise technique, improving overall eating patterns, exploring the possibility of an exciting career change, or embarking on a new relationship. Whatever we choose needs to include an element of fun and enjoyment or it becomes difficult to maintain enthusiasm: it is always much easier to stick to fresh intentions when they involve an activity that we enjoy.

Essential Energy

When we feel confident and at ease with ourselves, problems seem to bounce off us without leaving any tell-tale dents. However, when we feel insecure and low, all it takes is for a slight knock to plunge us into the depths of self-doubt and self-criticism. The latter situation often follows on from a period of low energy where we just don't feel we have the emotional or physical resilience to bounce back. This results in a downward spiral which lowers our energy resources even further, so that we have even fewer reserves with which to fight back if we're feeling low.

When energy reserves are high we can fight off infection, feel wide awake and vital through our working day, have extra bounce to feel alert in the evening, and have the enthusiasm to make time for regular exercise (which further boosts our energy levels). High energy levels are also essential to creative impulses, whether these are expressed through writing, dancing, singing, making love, or whatever.

As part and parcel of improved energy levels, we also experience clarity of mind, which aids the creative flow of ideas. Conversely, low energy levels are almost always accompanied by sluggish mental processes and indecision. Sustained vital energy makes our eyes sparkle, our hair shine and our skin look clear and vibrant. Most important of all, healthy, steady levels of energy give us a glow which communicates dynamism and vitality: attributes which are arguably the most attractive of all.

Vital energy flows most smoothly when we are at peace with ourselves: when the opposite is true we feel at odds with ourselves and the world at large. This does not, however, need to be as random as it sounds: there are ways of managing situations that deplete our stores of energy and those that boost and protect vitality. Some of these methods have already been mentioned in detail, for example, exercise, nutrition and dynamic systems of medicine such as homoeopathy; but there are important additional energy boosters and depleters which are outlined below.

Energy Wasters

Anxiety
Although summed up in a single word, anxiety describes a state that can vary from the mildest symptoms of unease to a severely disabling condition which can make life almost unbearable. Common symptoms of anxiety include:

• Palpitations.

• Dizziness.

• Sweating.

• Nausea or vomiting.

• Trembling.

• Panic.

• Breathlessness.

We need to differentiate between the sort of anxiety which is a perfectly appropriate response to a threatening situation and long-term anxiety in which we may experience diffused and enervating feelings. A good example of the former would be anxiety that comes from being in direct physical danger, such as being confronted by a ferocious bull in a field who is about to take a run at us. In this situation, feeling anxiety and fear is essential, otherwise we would not experience the bodily changes that are necessary for escape. When exposed to a threatening situation our bodies respond by secreting adrenalin, circulation is diverted away from digestive organs to our muscles, our hearts beat faster, and our blood pressure rises. As a result of these processes we are able to remove ourselves from the physical threat with ease and increased speed.

As you can see, anxiety reactions in the above context are essential to our survival. However, the same reaction when experienced on a low-grade, long-term basis is no longer appropriate or helpful. In other words, if we experience the same reactions in a milder form every time we are faced with a stressful situation, we can end up with long-term digestive problems, palpitations, high blood-pressure, and chronically low energy levels. This gets even more complicated when everyday situations such as receiving a bill or hearing the telephone ring are interpreted as threatening or stressful and result in elevated levels of adrenalin.

One of the ways of combating this vicious cycle is by exercising on a regular basis, since this can diffuse stressful situations by releasing endorphins and providing an escape-route for excess adrenalin. Most important of all, exercising regularly helps boost our energy levels and speed up our metabolic rate. This is particularly important when we consider how long-term anxiety compromises many of the benefits of vital energy. These include:

- Sleeping soundly.

- Increased concentration and clarity of thought.

- Efficient and trouble-free digestion.

- Clear and healthy skin.

- The ability to relax and unwind.

There are several constructive steps we can take to combat long-term anxiety and contribute to high energy levels, including:

- Keeping stimulants in the diet to a minimum; especially strong tea, coffee and caffeinated drinks.

- Avoiding reliance on sugary foods in order to keep going.

- Learning how to relax by using relaxation techniques, Yoga, or aromatherapy oils.

- Taking time out to have a massage or long soak in a relaxing scented bath.

- Taking up a regular form of exercise that is fun and enjoyable.

- Exploring breathing techniques.

- Using an alternative medical system such as homoeopathy, herbalism or acupuncture for long-term help with the problem.

- Having counselling or psychotherapy if you feel anxiety is beginning to be a regular and disabling feature of your life.

Depression

As with anxiety, there are varying types and degrees of depression that need to be identified if we are to put individual cases into context.

Depression can fall into two main categories: **reactive** or **endogenous**. The former is the sort of low feeling that we will all have felt from time to time: this can follow on from the break-up of a relationship, an unhappy work situation, or the loss of a close friend or relative; in other words, 'reacting' to an identifiable trigger. Once the situation has been resolved, reactive depression fades away, and does not usually return until another stressful or sad event comes around. Endogenous depression, on the other hand, needs no specific event to set it off. It 'grows from inside'. It can seem to descend out of the blue for no obvious reason, and can last for a protracted period. Because of its random, long-term nature, depression of this kind can be both exhausting and frightening, and very difficult to deal with for both sufferer or close family and friends.

Clearly, this level of depression needs help from experienced practitioners who are familiar with the usual course of the problem and who are able to help with the despair that can be a central part of it. Possible treatment options include: psychotherapy, psychiatric help, and orthodox drugs such as antidepressants or tranquillizers if, as is common, depression is accompanied by anxiety. Alternative medical options can also be of tremendous help in dealing with depression because of the emphasis which is put on evaluating the links between state of mind and physical symptoms. For those who are unhappy about the potential side-effects of antidepressants or the addictive problem associated with the use of tranquillizers, this can provide a valuable alternative.

Possible symptoms of depression include:

- Feelings that life is worthless or meaningless.

- Loss of confidence or self-esteem.

- Anxiety and panic attacks.

- Mood swings and erratic behaviour.

- Sleep disturbance.

- Lack of energy.

- Confusion and lethargy.

- Loss of libido.

- Digestive problems.

- Headaches.

- Skin rashes and irritation.

Since anxiety and depression are often related problems and overlap frequently, some of the symptoms in the anxiety section are also relevant to depression. The following suggestions will be helpful if you are experiencing transient depression of a reactive nature: if the problem is more long-term and you suspect it is of the endogenous variety these measures may still be of use, but you should also seek advice and assessment of a professional nature rather than dealing with the situation on your own.

- Check your diet and try to eliminate or cut down on foods that may intensify changes of mood, for example:

  - Chocolate.

  - Strong coffee.

  - Alcohol.

  - Sugar.

  - Wheat.

Foods to concentrate on are those that provide you with essential vitamins and minerals. These include as much fresh, raw fruit and vegetables as possible, fish, chicken, and dairy products in moderation. Also, try to drink plenty of mineral water and experiment with caffeine-free hot drinks such as herb teas or coffee substitutes.

- If you feel depressed because of a specific problem or worry, try not to dwell on it by yourself. Talk things over with a close friend or anyone you feel you trust and are at ease with. Gaining perspective on a problem can help enormously: once your feelings about a difficult situation have been verbalized they often become much less threatening.

- If there is no one you can talk to, write down your feelings and make a list of pros and cons of different ways of dealing with it.

- Don't feel guilty if you want to cry, or just can't stop crying. It is far better to express emotions when they surface rather than feeling you need to keep a stiff upper lip. The latter can lead to long-term problems that are related to unexpressed emotions, such as unexplained feelings of resentment or unhappiness.

- Organize a special treat for yourself: this can be anything that you know you enjoy and which cheers you up Make the range as wide as possible and use your imagination. Possibilities include:

  - Go away for a day or weekend with a friend or on your own to a place that you love.

  - Take time off in which to rest and have some space to yourself.

• Book yourself in for a massage, facial or range of treatments that make you feel pampered.

• Spend an evening watching your favourite videos, listening to your favourite music, or reading a novel you may not have had time to read.

• Use aromatherapy oils to help you relax or increase your sense of well-being. You can use these on a lamp burner, or put a few drops on your pillow, or add a small quantity to your bathwater. Remember to use them sparingly: use no more than two to four drops. Possibilities include: Geranium, Neroli, Nutmeg, Jasmine, Rose or Ylang Ylang.

• If you are not getting much exercise, make a point of increasing physical activity. Regular, aerobic exercise is a powerful way of improving sensations of well-being on both emotional and physical levels. You don't have to run a marathon, just make time to walk regularly, take the stairs rather than the lift, and avoid using transport to destinations that can easily be reached on foot.

Stress

Stress in itself need neither be pernicious or destructive: it is the way in which we perceive and respond to stress that determines its effect on us. It often helps to differentiate between positive and negative stress. Positive stress is the short-term variety caused by something demanding such as an examination or deadline. This is the sort of stress that gets us motivated and moving so that we perform well for the task in hand, and then allows us to relax when the demand has been met. Feeling under pressure in these circumstances makes our minds sharper and our responses swifter, sensations that can be further heightened by the knowledge that once the task has been achieved or the deadline met, we can enjoy a very necessary period of relaxation.

Negative stress, on the other hand, is more long-term and can often be experienced as a slow sensation of mental and physical tension which can erupt at intervals into feelings of blind panic or irritability. This form of stress is the opposite of that outlined above: it is fundamentally counterproductive, since it impairs and muddies mental processes, thus making decisions much more difficult to take. All of the following can be symptoms of feeling stressed:

• Mental and physical sensations of unease and tension.

• Insomnia.

• Irritability and anxiety.

• Feeling overwhelmed by even the smallest of tasks.

• Palpitations.

- Panic attacks.

- Relying on stimulants such as coffee to keep going, and cigarettes to relax.

- Nausea, heartburn and indigestion.

- Constipation and/or diarrhoea.

- Poor-quality skin.

- Migraines.

- Lack of energy.

In many ways, long-term, counterproductive stress is one of vitality's greatest enemies, since it depletes our energy level without our even being aware of it. In the same way that long-term pain or anxiety leaves us feeling shattered, feeling under stress produces a similar reaction. Because it is difficult to eat well when feeling under strain, this compounds the problem since at these times it is essential to have a plentiful supply of the nutrients that support our nervous system, such as the B vitamins or the mineral magnesium.

Other related problems include the likelihood of constipation from a diet lacking in fibre, constant indigestion and acidity from the inclusion of 'quick fix' foods, the effects of smoking and over-consumption of alcohol, and lack-lustre hair, skin, eyes and nails from a combination of all these factors. If we add into the equation additional problems of insomnia and aches in muscles and joints from constant muscular tension, clearly stress

of this kind is one of the major obstacles preventing us from looking and feeling on top form.

There are, however, a wide range of positive steps you can take to help you manage the stress levels in your life, rather than feeling that stress manages you.

Identify a list of priorities for yourself so that tasks that require immediate attention can be dealt with first, and less pressing jobs can be put off until a less stressful time. This will help you to work out what areas of stress in your life can be eliminated or reduced to a manageable level.

Although it sounds very obvious, making a list in this way can stop you feeling as though you can't work out what on earth needs tackling first. When these feelings of being bogged down occur we are left feeling stressed-out and confused, so that very often nothing gets done and we are left feeling even more tense and guilty.

Putting the tasks you need to tackle on paper immediately makes them less threatening and things that require immediate priority tend to stand out. Writing things out also has the important effect of focusing the mind, helping us to think more clearly about matters in hand.

Organize your surroundings. In many ways our external environment can reflect our state of mind: in other words, it is very easy to feel overwhelmed by what we have to do when we are surrounded by clutter. Conversely, once we start to organize our work or home surroundings work becomes much easier to come to grips with. On a practical level, pieces of paper in a file are much faster and easier to locate than those that are buried in a bottomless heap; finding them easily results in much less frustration and irritation. As always, however, the question of balance needs to be considered, since it is possible for a preoccupation with neatness to become a prison if it gets to the point of an obsession, in which case maintaining order can take over from the work itself, since all the effort is put into preparing for work rather than doing it.

Provided keeping order is seen as no more than a helpful and flexible tool which assists us in getting down to work more easily, it can be of immense value in diffusing stress and preventing us putting things off indefinitely.

Delegate as much as possible. This can be one of the side benefits of putting tasks on paper, since that often makes it clear that many of the things that need to be done can be handled perfectly well by someone else. Becoming aware of this and asking for help can be immensely liberating. It is also helps us discover that we are not as indispensable as we thought. Once learnt, delegating can reduce stress levels almost overnight.

Change your eating pattern. The digestive problems that come with a stressed lifestyle can be kept to a minimum if you make a few adjustments to your diet. These are foods that commonly contribute to indigestion and which should therefore be kept to a minimum:

- Fatty foods such as full-fat cheese, red meat, and rich sauces.

- Onions.

- Hot peppers.

- Very spicy dishes such as chillies and hot curries.

- Strong coffee or tea.

In addition it is best to avoid eating on the run, or when you feel tense or upset: digestion is always likely to happen more easily and smoothly if you can take time to relax and enjoy what you're eating.

One of the major problems of a stressed lifestyle is constipation, which can make anyone look and feel wretched. Keeping levels of fibre in the diet high, drinking 4–5 glasses of mineral water daily, and avoiding processed food are all simple ways of avoiding the problem.

Exercise can also be an invaluable tool in diffusing stress and tension, but it is important to stress that you should avoid falling into the trap of taking up a form of exercise that is very competitive, since this can result in making you feel even more tense.

Whatever form of exercise you choose needs to be fun and conducive to helping you relax and unwind afterwards: if you feel even more strung-out after exercising, the chances are that you need to look elsewhere. If you have found the best form of activity for yourself, you should find that your mind can switch off easily before sleep, and your body should feel relaxed and at ease. Systems of exercise which claim to encourage relaxation include Yoga, Medau, and the Pilates technique.

Breathing and relaxation techniques or meditation can also be of enormous help in trying to reduce stress levels. To achieve a meditative state, sit in a comfortable chair in a quiet room, making sure you keep your spine straight. Try to empty your mind of stressful or distracting thoughts by focusing on an image, either something in front of you or just a mental picture. You can try, if you prefer, to close your eyes and repeat a sound to yourself over and over again; this could be as simple as repeating the word 'one' or any other sound that appeals to you as you observe and regulate your breathing pattern. If you find distracting thoughts entering your mind, gently push them aside and refocus your attention on your chosen image or sound.

Set aside time for yourself every day, away from the demands of others. This is perhaps the most important way of reducing stress that we have at our disposal. It need be no more than five or ten minutes when you are very busy, or as long as half an hour or an hour when you can set aside the time. Whatever your resources, make this a time when

you can choose to do whatever helps you to relax and feel refreshed. This could be anything that suits you as an individual: soaking in a bath, having a walk in the fresh air, listening to music, or sitting for a while and doing absolutely nothing.

You can also use any of the suggestions from the section on Anxiety (above, p.160) that appeal to you, especially if you start to feel panicky when feeling tense.

Addiction

Although we often think automatically of drug dependence when we consider the question of addiction, this is a much broader phenomenon and can include dependence on chocolate, sugar, alcohol, coffee, dieting, exercise, playing computer games or even watching television. Once you become dependent on any of these to get through the day, and feel seriously threatened at the thought that any of them might be withdrawn, the chances are that an addictive state has developed, which may be physical and/or emotional.

It is obviously necessary to get things in perspective by differentiating between addictions that can be life-threatening, such as dependence on hard drugs or alcohol, those that can be seriously disruptive of family life and relationships, such as addiction to exercise, and those with less serious consequences such as a craving for chocolate or panicking and feeling anxious at the thought of missing a favourite television programme. It is, however, essential to appreciate that

167

addictive behaviour can seriously compromise our energy levels, leaving us feeling wrung out until we can have our next 'fix' of sugar, coffee, alcohol, cigarettes, or chocolate. After an initial boost of energy or mental stimulation, we are left back at square one again, needing further amounts of whatever we crave to maintain a feeling of well-being.

In order to highlight how enormous the issue of addiction is, these are just some of the substances and activities that can lead to addictive behaviour:

• Compulsive exercising.

• Falling in love.

• Workaholism.

• Shopping.

• Compulsive eating and/or dieting.

• Obsessions with cleaning and washing.

• Cigarettes.

• Prescription and recreational drugs.

• Alcohol.

• Sugar.

• Coffee and tea.

• Salt.

• Chocolate.

Apart from the common feature of gratification that all of the above supply, there is a further common link shared by many: falling in love, regular aerobic exercise, drinking alcohol, taking drugs such as cocaine and amphetamines, and making love all have biochemical effects on the body, resulting in ecstatic and stress-relieving sensations. These sensations are linked to the release of opioids, such as endorphins and enkephalins. Because these sensations are so pleasurable, it is possible to develop a habit of relying on them or turning to chocolate, alcohol, or cigarettes every time we feel down or stressed. Once this has been established as a pattern, being without our particular crutch in a period of stress can feel unbearable.

It obviously makes very little sense, then, to take the outmoded attitude that it only requires willpower to conquer an addiction. This view assumes that addiction is limited only to a psychological attachment, rather than involving a series of complex biochemical interactions which lead to physical cravings and extreme feelings of discomfort when the addictive substance is withdrawn. One of the worst aspects of the moralistic stance involved in the 'willpower' approach is the guilt that many people suffer on finding they cannot give up their addictive behaviour. Since common features suffered by those who have experienced addiction include fear, uncertainty, low self-esteem, and feelings of meaninglessness and powerlessness, adding feelings of guilt and failure to the equation is obviously unlikely to be helpful.

Common problems associated with addiction include the following:

- Permanently low or severely fluctuating energy levels.

- Difficulty with concentration.

- Severe mood swings.

- Irritability.

- Sleep disorders.

- Unstable weight patterns.

- Digestive problems.

- Low self-esteem.

- Feelings of anxiety.

- Depression.

- Headaches.

When we add into all this the fact that addiction to alcohol and/or cigarettes can also lead to illness and signs of premature ageing such as poor skin tone and texture, and that compulsive eating can also lead to weight gain and unhappiness with body image, the effects of addiction on both the physical and mental levels are multiplied.

There are a number of ways of helping ourselves through the maze of addiction:

- First of all, accept that you have a problem: many of us who are addicted will be very sensitive to criticism and become over-defensive, denying that there is a problem at all. Remember that without taking this difficult vital step it will be impossible to come to terms with your addiction.

- Support is essential if you are to succeed in giving up whatever you are addicted to. For instance, if you want to avoid alcohol, spend your time with friends who are happy to meet in surroundings other than a pub.

- Be willing to congratulate yourself as you make progress: find ways of rewarding yourself that bring you pleasure and boost your self-esteem.

- Identify the situations that most often are associated with a craving, such as knowing that when you get into work the first thing you do is light up a cigarette. If you are prepared for this you have a chance of finding a substitute, rather than feeling deprived or resentful and perhaps falling back into the habit.

- Be careful with cutting out coffee: if you are accustomed to drinking large quantities of strong coffee every day, you are likely to experience caffeine withdrawal. If this happens, be prepared for feeling generally listless and unwell, experiencing a severe headache, and feeling very on edge and irritable. If you want to avoid a severe reaction cut down systematically on your coffee intake, introducing enjoyable substitutes each day.

• If you have a lapse don't give up, but look at what you have achieved up to that point and just begin again.

• Consider getting help and support from groups that are specifically oriented towards assisting anyone who is struggling with addiction.

• Make sure you get the full range of vitamins and minerals you need from your diet. Concentrate on fresh fruit, green leafy vegetables, unsalted nuts, and sprouted or unsprouted seeds. Sunflower seeds can be especially valuable in keeping cravings for cigarettes at bay. Also ensure that you keep your blood sugar levels stable by eating at regular intervals rather than skipping meals.

Energy Boosters

The good news is that there are positive steps you can take to protect and boost your energy levels. By concentrating on the following when you start to feel your vitality flagging, you can ensure that you enjoy increased well-being as quickly as possible.

Eating for Energy

When feeling stressed or exhausted we can adopt ways of eating that are designed to counteract feeling woolly-headed or sluggish: ensuring that you eat small quantities regularly to maintain steady blood sugar levels, for example. Fruit is excellent since it contains fructose (fruit sugar) which does not wreak the same havoc as sucrose (table sugar) in the bloodstream. Other possibilities would include raw vegetables such as carrot sticks or celery which you can prepare in advance, or oat or rice cakes with whatever topping you choose. Avoid the following since they will only make you feel more depleted of energy in the long-run:

• Biscuits and cakes made from refined sugar and flour.

• Chocolate.

• Sweetened drinks such as fruit squashes or carbonated drinks.

• Coffee.

• Fatty foods which are difficult to digest such as hard cheese, foods with rich, creamy sauces, or meats such as pork or bacon.

• Alcohol.

• Chemically preserved foods with a high proportion of additives such as dehydrated snack foods.

If you feel that you have been experiencing acutely low energy levels as a result of over-indulgence in food and alcohol over a long period of time (such as over the Christmas period), you may benefit from following a fruit fast for a day or two. This should only be considered if you are in good health and provided you do not suffer from a medical condition such as diabetes. If in doubt about whether you should consider this or not, consult your GP or qualified alternative practitioner about the suitability and safety of fasting.

Stimulating and Protecting the Lymph System

We are dependent on the efficient flow of lymph through our bodies in order to remove toxins from our systems, to transport nutrients into our tissues, and above all, to help our immune systems to work smoothly and efficiently. There are excellent reasons for supporting and protecting our lymphatic systems:

• Because our immune systems are dependent upon the smooth working of the lymphatic system, keeping the latter in good order helps guard against disease and recurrent infections.

• Doing so prevents fatigue and lethargy.

• It will protect us from signs of early ageing as a result of cell degeneration.

• It will minimize the risk of developing cellulite.

When we consider how dependent we are on our lymphatic system for feeling and looking good, it makes very good sense to take constructive and positive steps to improve its function. Skin brushing, for example, is one of the most straightfor-ward, effective and simple ways of

encouraging lymphatic drainage. You will need to use a natural bristle brush with which to brush your skin: use sweeping movements which cover your body, moving downwards to the trunk and upwards from the feet to the legs and hips. The pressure you use should not be too vigorous at first, especially if you are not very fit: just use a degree of pressure that feels comfortable to you. You only need to go over your body once a day for optimum effect in eliminating toxic waste through the skin and stimulating lymphatic drainage.

Dealing With Cellulite
You will also find that skin brushing is one of the most effective allies you can have in dealing with cellulite: the bumpy-looking skin that settles on hips, thighs, arms, and stomach, and that resembles orange peel. The pitted appearance of the skin reveals that the tissues have become stagnant, holding on to toxic waste due to poor circulation and inefficient flow of lymph.

Cellulite is not just a cosmetic nuisance; its presence is also a physical indication that our systems are not eliminating wastes from our bodies as efficiently as they should. The result of this situation is the accompanying lethargy and lassitude that accompany the presence of cellulite.

Other ways of diminishing cellulite include:

• Regular, low-intensity aerobic exercise which is enjoyed three to five times a

171

week. This stimulates circulation, increases the capacity of the body to take in and utilize oxygen, and stimulates the flow of lymph. All of these are vital to any plan which aims to reduce cellulite. The exercise you choose depends on your personality and what appeals to you as individual: consider cycling, skiing, rowing, dancing, brisk walking, or swimming. The length of time you spend exercising should leave you feeling mentally and physically stimulated, not exhausted, and you must aim at regular rather than erratic exercise patterns. For instance, it is better to aim for twenty minutes physical activity three or four times a week than two hours every fortnight.

- Avoid cellulite-encouraging foods including dairy products with a high proportion of animal fat, red meat, refined sugar, junk foods (including pre-cooked meals), coffee, tea, salt, and alcohol. Foods that help fight cellulite include whole grains, large helpings of fresh fruit and vegetables, fish, additive-free poultry and eggs, and as much mineral water as possible. Kelp and seaweeds also have a part to play in dealing with cellulite production. You should always eat regularly and slowly, ensuring that you take time to chew adequately in order to help the process of digestion.

- Avoid crash dieting: apart from undermining overall vitality and encouraging exhaustion, extreme weight-loss plans usually do nothing to help stabilize weight at a healthy

level. In fact, those who are constantly dieting usually find that the pounds that have been shed usually return very speedily once they start eating normally again.

A vicious circle of weight loss and weight gain can encourage cellulite deposits because crash dieting encourages the breaking down of muscle tissue in the body, replacing it with fatty tissue which contributes to the formation of cellulite. Being on a severely restricted diet which emphasizes counting calories at the expense of the quality of food eaten also deprives the body of basic nutrients which are required to prevent or arrest cellulite production.

- Avoid baths that are very hot and very tight clothes which are restrictive of circulation: both can contribute to cellulite.

Lymphatic Drainage Massage is also claimed to be an effective way of helping stimulate our lymph systems, thus aiding in reduction of cellulite. Other conditions that may benefit from lymphatic drainage massage include water retention, spotty skin, muscle tension, low resistance to illness, and general lethargy and tiredness. Lymphatic massage stimulates the flow of blood and lymph through slow pumping movements, thus aiding the body in its cleansing and detoxifying functions.

Breathing for Purity
As we have seen in the previous chapter, by learning to breathe from the abdomen

(diaphragm) it is possible to feel calmer, more relaxed and less tense; diaphragmatic breathing also results in a sensation of invigoration, increased clarity of mind, and improved energy levels. Apart from these vital roles, breathing also performs a larger role than we might imagine in basic cleansing and the elimination of toxic waste from our bodies. The section 'First Steps in Breathing Technique' (p.112) describes how to breathe correctly for increased health, vitality and well-being.

Other possible variations on abdominal breathing include inhaling for a count of four, holding the breath gently for a count of four, and exhaling for a count of four. This cycle can be repeated for up to ten repetitions of the cycle, depending on when you feel you need to stop. The important thing is to feel relaxed and comfortable, avoiding any sense of strain.

You can also experiment with alternate nostril breathing. This is a breathing technique used in Yoga which can be helpful if you suffer from insomnia or general feelings of tension. Inhale through one nostril for a count of four, close both nostrils while you hold your breath gently for a count of four, exhale through the opposite nostril and pause for a final count of four before you begin the cycle again, inhaling through the nostril you have just exhaled from. Breathe slowly and gently without straining: you may find it easier to concentrate on maintaining a smooth breathing pattern if you close your eyes while you are going through this breathing exercise.

Consciously expel as much air as possible when you exhale to enable optimum use of each fresh inhalation into your lungs. By emptying your lungs more fully, you will increase the amount of carbon dioxide which is exhaled, and rid yourself of a larger proportion of waste products. Few of us breathe to our full capacity, which means that we are depriving our skin cells of essential oxygen. As a result, cell division is impeded: without the smooth functioning of this process the elimination of waste matter is compromised, leading to early ageing of these tissues.

Invigorating Body Treats

Hydrotherapy

Water is such a basic element in our lives that it is very easy for us to take it for granted. We can survive without food for a surprisingly long period of time, but if we are deprived of water we will die very rapidly. Dehydration happens rapidly in illness when, for example, vomiting and diarrhoea occur simultaneously, a condition which can be fatal if not arrested in time.

Our affinity with this element should hardly be surprising if we consider that our bodies are made up of more than 70 per cent water. We depend upon the free circulation of this basic liquid for the maintaining of basic body functions. Without water we stop eliminating wastes from our bodies, with the fatal consequence of a build-up of toxic matter.

While water plays an essential role in our survival on a physiological level, therefore, it can also have a very positive effect on both mind and body when applied within the context of hydrotherapy.

The use of water as a basic element in the process of healing is not new: spa towns in Britain and Europe based their claims for success on the therapeutic effects of 'taking the waters'. Spa water was believed to have positive effects, when taken internally or when bathed in, for a range of disorders which affected the skin and internal organs alike.

Although many of the spa resorts in popular use today use sea water treatments (Thalassotherapy), the use of fresh water for its healing properties (Hydrotherapy) was developed by Sebastian Kneipp in the nineteenth century. The techniques developed by Kneipp are still in use today in European hospitals and spa resorts, and it is claimed that they improve sluggish circulation, increase vitality, help protect against illness and improve skin condition. Hydrotherapy is hailed today as an important ally in fighting cellulite, and it may bring other advantages, such as:

- Improved mucous membrane function and reduction in catarrh as more toxins are eliminated through the skin rather than the mucous membranes.

- Better lung, kidney, and bowel action as the skin takes on a more eliminative function.

- Improvement in skin colour and tone.

It is possible to utilize some of Kneipp's techniques at home, but you should only consider doing so if you are in excellent health with no serious health problems such as circulatory disorders, diabetes, or a very inflamed skin disorder. If in doubt, always consult your GP, homoeopath, or another qualified practitioner before embarking on any course of action you may be unsure about. If you choose to try hydrotherapy at home, observe the following:

- Never apply cold water to your skin if you are chilled. Make sure you are warm by taking a warm shower or exercising gently first. You do not need to use cold water for more than thirty seconds.

- If you are unsure about using cold water on its own, start by using warm water and alternate with cold.

- After you have finished, leave areas to dry naturally rather than towelling off your whole body. Only dry those areas that will not be covered by clothing.

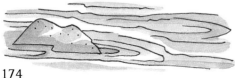

- Generate body warmth after cold treatments by going for a brisk, short walk. You can also choose to rest in bed after a warm treatment.

Hydrotherapeutic treatments at spa resorts use high-power water jets. These are directed at specific areas of the body, such as the buttocks, hips, and thighs in an effort to speed-up circulation. You can imitate this technique by using a hand-held shower.

- Begin by taking a warm shower. Switch to cold for about twenty seconds, back to warm, and finally cold again.

- To increase vitality you can move down the body starting with your face, moving down your arms and legs, to your chest, stomach, and finally down your back.

- You can utilize cold water treatments for a specific part of the body in order to tone up the quality of the skin. A good example would include spraying your breasts with cold water in order to preserve the firmness or smoothness of the skin. Other techniques to consider include using two flannels: one resting in a bowl of cold water and the other in hot water. Apply the hot flannel which has been wrung out to one breast until it is fully warmed. Follow this with the cold flannel which has been wrung out in the same way. Concentrate on one breast at a time, using three applications of hot and cold, always ending with cold.

Bathing

Taking baths can be a way of encouraging relaxation, resting the body, and soothing tired and aching muscles. Luxuriating in a warm, scented bath does not have the invigorating effect of a shower, but it can have a large part to play in aiding detoxification as well as relaxing mind and body. To get the maximum benefit from your bath, try the following:

- Add to your bathwater essential oils which complement your mood. Consider Lavender, Vetiver, Chamomile, Rose or Geranium as soothing bath essences. If you want a stimulating or uplifting bath, consider Sandalwood, Tangerine or Neroli. Remember to use them sparingly.

- Make sure your bathwater is warm, not hot: the ideal temperature should not exceed 97–100°F (36–38°C); otherwise you are likely to feel enervated rather than refreshed afterwards. Other problems which can result from too hot a bath include raised blood pressure and over dilated blood capillaries.

- Use an exfoliating cream on damp skin over hips, thighs, knees, elbows, and heels before getting into your bath, or apply the exfoliator after you have finished soaking in the bath.

- Consider using seaweed preparations in your bathwater, or applying a mud treatment before showering. Both seaweed and mud are considered to have detoxifying and cleansing qualities when applied to the skin. Make sure that your bathwater is no hotter than tepid or warm if you are using seaweed: a hot seaweed bath will make your heart rate speed up uncomfortably.

Saunas

Saunas are well known for raising body temperature and encouraging perspiration, thus enabling the body to eliminate toxins more efficiently through the skin. Other possible beneficial effects of taking a sauna include increased sensations of vitality, improved skin texture, and a feeling of mental calmness.

If you are taking any prescription drugs or if you suffer from any of the following, you should avoid using a sauna unless your GP has advised you to the contrary:

- Heart disease or general circulatory disorders.

- Serious problems with breathing such as asthma or emphysema.

- High temperature or any acute illness.

In any event, there are certain guidelines you should follow if you are taking a sauna, especially if you are unfamiliar with what to expect:

- Take things very easily: do not feel you have to stay in the heat for longer than you feel comfortable. As soon as you feel you have had enough or you begin to feel light-headed or dizzy, come out of the sauna, have a cool shower and rest until you feel ready to begin again.

- Try to lie down with as little covering your body as possible in order to gain maximum benefit from the heat. Make sure you have removed any metal jewellery from your body, since this will become very hot.

- At first restrict yourself to staying on the lower benches; only move to the higher ones when you are familiar with how you respond to the heat.

- Avoid taking a sauna immediately after a meal or if you have been feeling unwell.

- Guard against dehydration by drinking plenty of water when you feel you need it.

- Make sure you leave enough time to rest at the end rather than rushing off immediately after you have finished your sauna. Allow yourself at least thirty minutes in which to unwind, relax, and feel the full benefit of the sauna treatment.

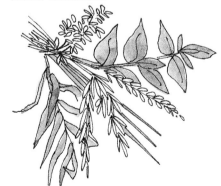

Appendix:

Homoeopathy in Action

ere are some examples of homoeopathic cases. They show how homoeopaths try to make sense of the symptoms their patients report, and how the information gathered on the initial visit can guide them to the appropriate first prescription. Most of all, these cases will highlight the essential importance of making the links between symptoms in order to understand how illness has developed. In this process it is inevitable that as much weight will be put on emotional as physical symptoms.

Case 1

Sarah was a young woman of 25 who came for homoeopathic treatment for pre-menstrual migraines, which she had experienced for two years. They had increased in severity, and any drugs she had used had not relieved her symptoms. She experienced excruciating pain with her migraine every month without fail, and felt it had reached the point where it dominated her life.

Her periods had always been difficult, mainly because she experienced marked irritability and tearfulness beforehand. Once the period arrived, these symptoms improved dramatically. When feeling down she needed a lot of space to herself, and could not abide sympathy or people fussing over her.

She experienced excellent health as a child, but felt herself begin to go down-hill in her teens. At this time she developed a very itchy patch of eczema on her leg. This disappeared after a steroid cream was applied. Her skin was generally very sensitive, with a particular tendency to flare up in an itchy rash if exposed to the sun. In the winter she would also expect to develop at least one or two cold sores. Over the next few years she noticed that she was beginning to develop hay-fever symptoms, which were treated by anti-histamines during the hay-fever season.

In her late teens the mood swings before her periods became more noticeable, but she had not felt any need to seek help from her doctor. The year before her migraines appeared her father died suddenly. Although her family was not an emotionally demonstrative one, she was especially close to her father and his death was a terrible shock to her. At the time of his death, and in the months following, she did not feel she could cry or show any outward sign of grieving; most of her time was occupied with caring for other members of her family, for whom she felt responsible. Although she had a small circle of friends, she had never talked with them about her father or how she had felt since his death.

Her energy levels were low most of the time, and she often craved stimulants in order to keep her going. Her favourite foods were salty, especially crisps and salted nuts.

On the basis of this information, *Natrum mur* was selected as the homoeopathic remedy most suited to her symptom picture as a whole. After a few months of treatment her migraines were not as severe, and with each episode they were getting shorter. Her energy levels improved, and she began to talk more about her grief for her father with each visit.

Within another short interval her migraines had gone, although she might experience the odd headache if she was exposed to sunlight for too long. After the interval of one year she returned with an eruption on her leg which she thought might be the return of her eczema, although it was not so large or severely

itchy. After a repeat dose of *Natrum mur* the eczema cleared up.

The days leading up to her period are no longer traumatic and her energy levels remain high provided she eats well and rests when she needs to. She still needs some homoeopathic help with her hay fever symptoms, but with each succeeding year her symptoms are diminishing in frequency and intensity. Now she no longer uses anti-histamines, but finds that when the symptoms are troublesome the homoeopathic remedy *Apis mel* makes her comfortable within a short space of time.

This case demonstrates beautifully the relationship between emotional and physical symptoms, and also how symptoms can become more complicated when suppressed. Neither the steroid cream nor the anti-histamines cured her condition, but merely pushed the disorder into the body to cause problems at internal levels. This patient might have continued to 'get by' at this stage, but the death of her father provided the last straw. Her migraines represented her body's way of expressing distress, and, as a result, any homoeopathic prescription selected would have to be heavily weighted towards unexpressed grief as well as the physical symptoms. As it happens, *Natrum mur* is a suitable remedy for all of the following:

• Complaints from suppressed grief.

• Dislike of consolation.

- Inability to cry.

- Disinclination to share problems.

- Marked irritability before periods.

- Recurrent headaches which are worse before periods.

- Sensitivity to sunlight.

- Tendency to develop cold sores.

- Tendencies to skin rashes including prickly heat and eczema, hay fever and allergic rhinitis.

- Craving for salt.

It is noticeable that, as her migraines improved, her energy levels also increased. Most important of all, we should take note of the return of the eczema which had been suppressed, since this indicates that the disorder was being pushed once more on to the periphery of the body. There is every likelihood that as her hay fever improves, the eczema will make another brief reappearance

Case 2

Maggie was 34 years of age. She had a history of joint problems, which began when she was in her late 20s. The pain and swelling had been treated with anti-inflammatory medication which relieved the pain, but on her first appointment she complained of troublesome digestive symptoms. These symptoms included stomach burning and acidity on an almost permanent basis, which could only be relieved by sipping warm drinks. She felt so nauseated that she ended up vomiting, but this did nothing to relieve the stomach discomfort.

When her stomach was very disturbed she could also experience repeated bouts of diarrhoea which left her feeling exhausted. As a result, she felt very despondent when these symptoms were intense, to the point of believing nothing could be done for her.

What worried her most of all was that she had become increasingly anxious: something that had always been around in small measure from time to time, but which was now threatening to dominate her life. She needed to be in company most of the time in order to take her mind off how she felt, and found that she was most anxious in bed at night.

This anxiety was threatening to disrupt her career, which was most important to her. She was—and still is—a high-powered businesswoman who kept a very busy schedule and demanded a lot of herself. Now, with her increasing lack of confidence she felt her condition was threatening to destroy her career. Worst of all, she was becoming so self-critical she was beginning to check and re-check everything she did.

In appearance she was slim and very well dressed, and obviously spent a lot of time on how she looked. The notes she made for her initial interview were all meticulously written down and organized in advance. She had a mobile phone which she felt to be essential to keep in touch with what is going on, in order to give her a sense of control. Without this she felt threatened.

She was sleeping fitfully and felt her energy levels had plummeted: previously she would have described them as dynamic. She always felt cold and preferred a warm environment.

After this case was analysed, *Arsenicum album* was chosen as the most appropriate homoeopathic remedy at that stage. The following are key features of the condition for which this remedy is suitable:

- Tremendous anxiety and restlessness which is much worse at night.

- Fear that recovery will not be forthcoming.

- Fear of losing control.

- Excessive attention to detail and fastidiousness.

- Perfectionism.

- Burning pains that are relieved by warmth (eg burning pains in the stomach relieved by sips of warm drinks).

- Exhausting diarrhoea.

- Very chilly and generally better for warmth.

On further visits the same remedy was repeated with favourable results. She began to feel energized, more relaxed, and her sleeping pattern improved enormously. The burning in the stomach had become negligible, and the diarrhoea had ceased altogether.

Everything proceeded well until she returned with the news that her symptoms seemed to have changed direction. Now she was feeling so much better, she was beginning to burn the candle at both ends in order to catch up on the time she felt she had missed at work when feeling so ill. In order to keep up working long hours and socializing almost every night, she had begun to drink increasingly large quantities of black coffee to keep going, and her alcohol consumption had gone up. Her digestive symptoms had now changed to a condition of constipation which she put down to her irregular eating habits. She also reported feeling irritable and very short-tempered when tired, and felt that she was regularly experiencing hangover-type headaches.

At this stage it was clear that a change of remedy would be needed to match the new symptom picture that was emerging. The remedy chosen was *Nux vomica*, which matches the following symptoms:

- Irritability from over-tiredness.

- Reliance on stimulants to keep energy levels high.

- Workaholism.

- Constipation.

- Craving for coffee.

- Frequent headaches.

After the first dose of *Nux vomica* the change was dramatic: improvement took place on all levels and things proceeded well for some time, with the remedy being repeated when needed.

All went well until a further change occurred: this time there were no problems with digestion and anxiety, but the symptoms associated with her joint problems were becoming more noticeable. The joints of her hands, knees, and feet were very painful and stiff, especially on waking in the morning. However, once she got moving they would feel much better, and provided she did not overdo things they would be much easier by the end of the day. The next morning things would be back to square one, with relief being provided by a warm shower or bath. She noticed that she could sense if it was a wet, cold day even before she got out of bed since her joints would feel much worse.

At this stage, *Rhus tox* was given daily for a short period of time. The main symptoms covered by *Rhus tox* in this case are as follows:

- Severe joint pains that are much worse for immobility.

- Relief of joint pains by continued motion, provided it does not exhaust.

- Pains that are relieved by warm bathing.

- Severe aggravation of pains in cold, wet weather.

After repetition of this remedy when needed over a period of several weeks, the joint pains subsided. Now Maggie knows that she needs to return for treatment whenever she feels her renewed level of health is slipping, even if it is a small change in her experience of general well-being, such as partially reduced energy levels, or a more specific complaint such as a return of her joint pains.

As we can see, this case provides a different perspective in highlighting how the homoeopath must be ready to change the remedy in accordance with changes in symptoms. Unlike the first case where *Natrum mur* was the only remedy required over a long-term basis because the symptoms remained essentially those which were covered well by that single prescription, in the second case continuing with *Arsenicum album* would have been of little avail when it was obvious that *Nux vomica* was required.

In the second case we can also see the same basic process at work as in the first, as the disorder moves from emotional

181

and mental levels to the more peripheral area: in this case to the joints. The essential clue that this is a curative development is provided by the information that the patient was vastly improved with regard to her energy levels and was experiencing much less anxiety. When we take this information and combine it with observation of the improvement in her digestive symptoms, it is clear that symptoms are moving to the periphery.

Case 3

Sally sought homoeopathic help because of recurring problems with swollen glands, sore throats and generalized muscle aching. She was especially concerned about her overall condition and diminishing levels of vitality, because at the age of 38 she had just been promoted to a job which involved increased responsibility.

Her main problem was a lack of stamina on mental, emotional and physical levels. Every time she felt things were getting on top of her she would experience a slow-developing sore throat, which would quickly affect the glands in her neck. If the infection was very severe, it would lead to swelling and tenderness under her arms and would usually result in a chest infection. The latter would be productive, leading her to cough up large quantities of green phlegm. This was often accompanied by a severe head cold, with a thick, bland, green-coloured nasal discharge. Her nose would be very

blocked up at night, so that she would end up with a dry mouth in the morning as a result of breathing through her mouth. Most bouts of chest infections had led to courses of antibiotics which left her with a repeated tendency to thrush.

Normally of fairly average temperature, once she developed a sore throat she would feel very chilly, but was reluctant to stay indoors because she felt that fresh air was the only thing that cleared her head. Once she got back indoors, she would feel stuffed-up again, which often resulted in headaches. The muscle aches in her back, shoulders, arms and legs would also feel better for moving about, and generally were worse overnight when she was in bed.

Normally easy-going and someone who enjoyed good working relationships and a lively social life, once she felt ill Sally began to feel very tearful and quickly depressed. The only thing that seemed to help was the company of friends who would offer sympathy and distraction: once she was on her own things got steadily worse. If she had a good cry, she would generally feel better for it.

Apart from this pattern of recurring symptoms there was no other marked feature of ill health in her medical history.

On the basis of the above information, *Pulsatilla* was chosen as the appropriate homoeopathic prescription. Conditions helped by *Pulsatilla* include:

- Tendencies to glandular problems.

- Thick catarrhal discharges which are green and bland.

- Muscle aches which are worse for keeping still.

- Catarrhal conditions and headaches which are much worse for warm rooms.

- Desire for fresh air although chilly.

- Blocked-up nose leading to dry mouth.

- Very weepy with illness.

- Better for sympathy.

- Better after crying.

Because of her low level of vitality and her lack of ability to fight infections effectively, along with taking her homoeopathic remedy she also increased the level of vitamin C in her diet through supplementation and by eating more fresh green vegetables, salad and fruit. She also made a conscious effort to rest when she felt she needed to relax, and stopped taking work home with her.

She attended a chiropractor for a number of sessions since the aches in her shoulders were particularly noticeable. Once these were relieved she also decided to have a regular full body massage, as she found this was invaluable in helping her to relax.

The overall result was a marked improvement on all levels over the period of a year, with very few episodes of infection. Most important of all, when a sore throat did appear, it was short-lived and did not go down to her chest. Eventually she reached the point where she was having no more colds and sore throats than the average person. Her energy levels were also restored to a point where she felt she could enjoy her increased responsibility without strain.

Recommended Reading

General Titles

Callen, Karena. *Vitality: Elle Guide To Health And Beauty*. London, 1991.

Chaitow, Leon. *Clear Body Clear Mind: How To Be Healthy In A Polluted World*. London, 1990.

Coleman, Vernon. *The Health Crisis: Your Health In Crisis*. London, 1988.

Ehrenreich, John (ed.). *The Cultural Crisis of Modern Medicine*. New York, 1978.

Inglis, Brian. *The Diseases of Civilisation: Why We Need A New Approach To Medical Treatment*. London, 1981.

Kenton, Leslie. *Ultrahealth: The Positive Way To Vitality And Good Looks*. London, 1984.

Kenton, Leslie. *Ten Day Clean-Up Plan: De-Toxify Your Body for Natural Health and Vitality*. London, 1986.

Kenton, Leslie and Susannah. *Time Alive: The High-Energy Way To Good Health and Natural Beauty*. London, 1987.

Kenton, Leslie. *Cellulite Revolution: Six Steps To A New Body Ecology*. London, 1992.

Kenton, Leslie and Susannah. *Endless Energy: A Workbook For Dynamic Health And Personal Power*. London, 1993.

Melville, Arabella and Johnson, Colin. *Cured to Death: The Effects of Prescription Drugs*. London, 1982.

Meredith, Bronwen. *Stay Younger Longer*. London, 1984.

Oliver, Keith, and Peiser, Andrea, *How are You? Why Normal isn't Normal*. London 1991.

Payer, Lynn. *Medicine and Culture: Notions of Health and Sickness in Britain, the US, France, and West Germany*. London, 1989.

Payne, Dr. Mark. *Superhealth: The Complete Environmental Medicine Health Plan*. London 1992.

Phillips, Angela and Rakusen, Jill. *The New Our Bodies, Ourselves: A Health Book For And By Women*. London, 1989.

Ronsard, Nicole. *Beyond Cellulite*. London, 1992.

Salmon, J. Warren. *Alternative Medicines: Popular and Policy Perspectives*. London, 1985.

Stoppard, Miriam. *Every Woman's Lifeguide: How to achieve and maintain fitness, health and happiness in today's world.* London, 1982.

Vincenzi, Penny. *Cosmopolitan's Vital Health Guide.* London, 1982.

Werbach, Melvyn, R. *Third Line Medicine: Modern Treatment For Persistent Symptoms.* London, 1986.

Wormwood, Valerie Ann. *The Fragrant Pharmacy: A home and health care guide to aromatherapy and essential oils.* London, 1990.

Alternative Medicine

Castro, Miranda. *The Complete Homoeopathy Handbook: A Guide to Everyday Health Care.* London, 1990.

Castro, Miranda. *Homoeopathy for Mother and Baby: Pregnancy, Birth and the Post-Natal Year.* London, 1992.

Fulder, Steven. *The Handbook of Complementary Medicine.* London, 1984.

Fulder, Steven. *How to be a healthy patient: a holistic guide to medical treatment.* London, 1991.

Handley, Rima. *Homoeopathy for Women.* London, 1993.

Kaptchuk, Ted and Croucher, Michael. *The Healing Arts: A Journey Through the Faces of Medicine.* London, 1986.

Lockie, Dr Andrew. *The Family Guide to Homoeopathy: The Safe Form of Medicine.* London, 1989.

Lockie, Dr Andrew and Geedes, Dr Nicola. *The Women's Guide to Homoeopathy: The Natural Way to a Healthier Life for Women.* London, 1992.

MacEoin, Beth. *Homoeopathy.* London, 1992.

Richardson, Sarah. *New Ways to Health: A Guide to Homoeopathy.* London, 1988.

Scott, Julian and Susan. *Natural Medicine For Women: Drug-Free Healthcare for Women of All Ages.* London, 1991.

Stanway, Andrew, *Alternative Medicine: A Guide To Natural Therapies.* London, 1982.

Ullman, Dana. *Homoeopathy: Medicine for the 21st Century.* Berkeley, 1988.

Vithoulkas, George. *The Science of Homoeopathy.* London, 1986.

Vithoulkas, George. *A New Model of Health and Disease.* Berkeley, 1991.

Westcott, Patsy. *Alternative Health Care For Women.* London, 1987.

Exercise

Alexander, Tania. *No Sweat Fitness: The Everyday Guide To Healthy Living For The 90s.* Edinburgh, 1992.

Barker, Sarah. *The Alexander Technique: The Revolutionary Way to Use Your Body for Total Energy.* London, 1978.

Barlow, Wilfred. *The Alexander Principle.* London, 1975.

Berk, Lotte and Price, Jean. *The Lotte Berk Method of Exercise.* London, 1989.

Caplin, Carole. *Holistix: The Revolutionary New Approach To Looking And Feeling Great.* London, 1990.

Fonda, Jane. *Women Coming of Age.* London, 1985.

Jackson, Lucy. *Medau: The art of energy.* London, 1992.

Marshall, Lynn. *Keep Up With Yoga.* London, 1986.

Marshall, Lynn. *Wake Up To Yoga.* London, 1988.

O'Brien, Paddy. *A Gentler Strength: The Yoga book for women.* London, 1991.

Nutrition

Ballantine, Rudolph. *Diet and Nutrition: a holistic approach.* Pennsylvania, 1982.

Eyton, Audrey. *The Complete F-Plan Diet.* London, 1982.

Grant, Doris, and Joice, Jean. *Food Combining for Health: Don't Mix Foods That Fight, A New Look at the Hay System.* London, 1991.

Kano, Susan. *Never Diet Again: The flexible eating plan to help you stay slim without dieting.* London, 1989.

Kenton, Leslie. *Raw Energy.* London, 1986.

Mayes, Adrienne. *The Dictionary of Nutritional Health: A Guide to The Relation Between Diet and Health.* Wellingborough, 1986.

Mervyn, Leonard. *The Dictionary of Minerals: The Complete Guide to Minerals and Mineral Therapy.* Wellingborough, 1986.

Mervyn, Leonard. *The Dictionary of Vitamins: The Complete Guide to Vitamins and Vitamin Therapy.* Wellingborough, 1984.

Montignac, Michel. *Dine Out and Lose Weight.* London, 1991.

Wright, Celia. *The Wright Diet: Your personal plan for permanent weight loss.* London, 1989.

Relaxation

Benson, Herbert. *The Relaxation Response.* London, 1976.

Benson, Herbert. *Beyond the Relaxation Response.* London, 1985.

Chaitow, Leon. *Your Complete Stress-Proofing Programme.* London, 1986.

Horn, Sandra. *Relaxation: Modern Techniques for Stress Management.* London, 1986.

Kirsta, Alix. *The Book of Stress Survival: How to Relax and Live Positively.* London, 1986

Useful Addresses

Council for Complementary and
Alternative Medicine
179 Gloucester Place
London NW1 6DX
Tel: 071 724 9103

Institute for Complementary Medicine
Unit 4
Tavern Quay
Rope Street
Rotherhithe
London SE16
Tel: 071 237 5165

Natural Medicines Society
Edith Lewis House
Ilkeston
Derbyshire DE7 8EJ
Tel: 0602 329454

British Complementary
Medical Association
St Charles' Hospital
Exmoor Street
London W10 6DZ
Tel: 081 964 1206

General Council and Register of
Osteopaths
56 London Street
Reading RG1 4SQ
Tel: 0734 576585

British Chiropractic Association
Premier House
10 Greycote Place
London SW1P 1SB
Tel: 071 222 8866

British Acupuncture Association and
Register
34 Alderney Street
London SW1V 4EV
Tel: 071 834 1012

National Register of Hypnotherapists and
Psychotherapists
12 Cross Street
Nelson
Lancs BB9 7EN
Tel: 0282 699378

National Institute Of Medical Herbalists
9 Palace Gate
Exeter
Devon EX1 1JA
Tel: 0392 426022

British Society for Autogenic Training
and Therapy
101 Harley Street
London W1N 1DF
Tel: 071 935 1811

British Society for Nutritional Medicine
PO Box 3AP
London W1A 3AP
Tel: 071 436 8532

West London School of Therapeutic
Massage
41 St Luke's Road
London W11 1DD
Tel: 071 229 4672

International Federation of
Aromatherapists
Royal Masonic Hospital
Ravenscourt Park
London W6 0TN
Tel: 081 846 8066

The British Homoeopathic Association
27a Devonshire Street
London WC1N 3HZ
Tel: 071 935 2163

The Hahnemann Society
2 Powis Place
Great Ormond Street
London WC1N 1RJ
Tel: 071 837 3297

Society of Homoeopaths
2 Artizan Road
Northampton NN1 4HU
Tel: 0604 21400

British Wheel of Yoga
1 Hamilton Place
Boston Road
Sleaford
Lincs. NG34 7ES
Tel: 0529 306851

Society of Teachers of the Alexander
Technique
Suite 20
10 London House
266 Fulham Road
London SW10 9EL
Tel: 071 351 0828

Pilates
Body Maintenance
2nd Floor, Pineapple
7 Langley Street
Covent Garden
London WC2H 9JA
Tel: 071 379 6043

Medau Society
8b Robson House
East Street
Epsom
Surrey KT17 1HH
Tel: 0372 729056

Lotte Berk Studio
29 Manchester Street
London W1M 5PS
Tel: 071 935 8905

Index